Writing for Nursing and Midwifery Students

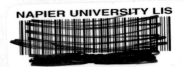

Palgrave Study Skills

Authoring a PhD
Business Degree Success
Career Skills
Critical Thinking Skills
e-Learning Skills (2nd edn)
Effective Communication for
  Arts and Humanities Students
Effective Communication for
  Science and Technology
The Exam Skills Handbook
The Foundations of Research
The Good Supervisor
How to Manage your Arts, Humanities and
  Social Science Degree
How to Manage your Distance and
  Open Learning Course
How to Manage your Postgraduate Course
How to Manage your Science and
  Technology Degree
How to Study Foreign Languages
How to Write Better Essays (2nd edn)
IT Skills for Successful Study
The International Student Handbook
Making Sense of Statistics
The Mature Student's Guide to Writing (2nd edn)
The Personal Tutor's Handbook
The Postgraduate Research Handbook (2nd edn)
Presentation Skills for Students

The Principles of Writing in Psychology
Professional Writing (2nd edn)
Researching Online
Research Using IT
Skills for Success
The Study Abroad Handbook
The Student's Guide to Writing (2nd edn)
The Student Life Handbook
The Study Skills Handbook (3rd edn)
Study Skills for Speakers of English as
  a Second Language
Studying the Built Environment
Studying Business at MBA and Masters Level
Studying Economics
Studying History (3rd edn)
Studying Law (2nd edn)
Studying Mathematics and its Applications
Studying Modern Drama (2nd edn)
Studying Physics
Studying Programming
Studying Psychology (2nd edn)
Teaching Study Skills and Supporting Learning
Work Placements – A Survival Guide for Students
Writing for Nursing and Midwifery Students
Write it Right
Writing for Engineers (3rd edn)

Palgrave Study Skills: Literature

General Editors: John Peck and Martin Coyle

How to Begin Studying English Literature
  (3rd edn)
How to Study a Jane Austen Novel (2nd edn)
How to Study a Charles Dickens Novel
How to Study Chaucer (2nd edn)
How to Study an E. M. Forster Novel
How to Study James Joyce
How to Study Linguistics (2nd edn)

How to Study Modern Poetry
How to Study a Novel (2nd edn)
How to Study a Poet
How to Study a Renaissance Play
How to Study Romantic Poetry (2nd edn)
How to Study a Shakespeare Play (2nd edn)
How to Study Television
Practical Criticism

Writing for Nursing and Midwifery Students

Julio Gimenez

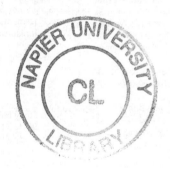

palgrave
macmillan

First published 2007 by
PALGRAVE MACMILLAN
Houndmills, Basingstoke, Hampshire RG21 6XS and
175 Fifth Avenue, New York, N.Y. 10010
Companies and representatives throughout the world

PALGRAVE MACMILLAN is the global academic imprint of the Palgrave
Macmillan division of St. Martin's Press, LLC and of Palgrave Macmillan Ltd.
Macmillan® is a registered trademark in the United States, United Kingdom
and other countries. Palgrave is a registered trademark in the European
Union and other countries.

ISBN-13: 978–0–230–00857–1
ISBN-10: 0–230–00857–7

This book is printed on paper suitable for recycling and made from fully
managed and sustained forest sources. Logging, pulping and manufacturing
processes are expected to conform to the environmental regulatons of the
country of origin.

A catalogue record for this book is available from the British Library.

10   9   8   7   6   5   4   3
16 15 14 13 12 11 10 09 08

Printed in China

Contents

List of Tables

List of Figures

Acknowledgements

My first debt of gratitude is to those who wrote about *writing* before me and have therefore influenced my views and approach to teaching how to write specific genres: John Swales, Charles Bazerman, Carolyn R. Miller, Chris Candlin, V.K. Bhatia and Ken Hyland, among many others.

I am also indebted to Suzannah Burywood, my commissioning editor at Palgrave Macmillan, for her support and encouragement. I would also like to thank the four reviewers of the book whose comments have made this a better project. I did not always follow their advice, however, so the remaining flaws are my entire responsibility.

I am thankful to my colleagues at Middlesex University who provided me with enlightening comments during the writing process. Special thanks go to Victoria Odeniyi and Gillian Lazar at ELLS. I am similarly grateful to Clare Maher and Jane Raymond for their invaluable comments and support with the discipline-specific contents of the book, and to Dilys Hall for introducing me to RefWorks. I am equally thankful to my colleague and friend Beverly Fairfax for her comments and feedback on the first draft of the book.

I am thankful to EndNote and RefWorks for permission to reproduce the screenshots on pages 117–4.

To my students past and present who have given me the best a teacher can get: challenging comments and questions. Most of the ideas and materials in this book started as answers to their questions.

These acknowledgements would be incomplete without thanking those who have been quietly waiting for the writing process to become a product; to Ines, Marianela and Facundo all my gratitude for their love and patience.

JULIO GIMENEZ

Introduction

● **About this book**

One of the most difficult tasks we are faced with when we enter university is *writing*. Not only are we asked to deal with new content, but we are also required to engage in new intellectual processes and, in many cases, we must even learn to organize and structure knowledge in new ways. Writing, and especially writing assignments, becomes even more taxing for adult students who have been away from formal education for quite some time and come back to university via top-up courses or 'back-to-practice' programmes.

This book has been designed and organized to help you with your writing tasks throughout your undergraduate programme. The book combines the theoretical approach of a textbook with the practical activities of a work-book.

Starting with the basic principles of writing at university level, the book first explores the generic essay, then analyses typical genres such as the care critique and the article review, and finally deals with argumentative writing and preparation for the undergraduate dissertation. The book includes authentic essay questions and examples at different levels of writing along with exercises on how to make writing in nursing and midwifery more effective.

The book also includes:

- ● an examination of different **referencing systems** such as the Harvard and the American Psychological Association (APA) styles;
- ● an introduction to the most common **bibliographic software** used at universities;
- ● a **glossary of key terms** that expands on the core concepts presented in the 'glossary boxes' in the book and that provides further examples;
- ● a list of **further readings and resources** that includes links to web-based materials;

- **suggested answers** to exercises, which will be very useful if you are working on your own;
- an **achievement chart** to help you keep a record of your progress.

What makes this book different

You will also find that the book is:

- **Specific** – it has been designed to meet the specific writing needs of student nurses and midwives. The book deals with the writing genres you will be asked to produce, from the academic and the reflective essay and the care critique to research proposals, reports and the dissertation;
- **Easy to use** – you will find that the 'how to' chapters cover all the main writing genres in a practical step-by-step way;
- **Active and engaging** – the chapters have been written in a very engaging style; reading them will not be a solitary activity, you will find a tutor at every step of the way;
- **Comprehensive** – in addition to the main writing genres, you will find a chapter on how to avoid plagiarism, one on how to use web-based bibliography managers, sample essay questions and how to answer them to meet typical marking criteria, and advice on grammar and language for the ESOL student;
- **Up-to-date** – the content is based on current theory and practice in nursing and midwifery and is aligned with the general bench-mark statements of international quality assurance associations.

I hope that by the end of the book you will feel more confident about writing in general, and writing the specific genres in nursing and midwifery in particular. Like any other type of writing, academic writing is a purposeful activity whose main aim is to satisfy the needs of its readers. And this is what I *really* hope this book will achieve.

JULIO C. GIMENEZ

Middlesex University

Part One

The Essentials of Academic Writing

The chapters in this part introduce you to the basics of writing in an academic environment, with a focus on your specific needs as a student of nursing or midwifery. You will first explore the principles of organizing and structuring information and see how these principles work for different kinds (and levels) of nursing and midwifery writing. You will then look at description and argumentation and how these can be put to work in different writing genres. Finally, you will examine more complex processes such as reflection and critical thinking.

• Chapter 1: An Introduction to Academic Writing

In this first chapter, you will find the essentials of academic writing at university level. The chapter starts by exploring background (what), rationale (why) and signposting (how) in essay planning. It then introduces the principles of 'macro structuring'. It will show you how to expand the structure of a paragraph into an essay, organize information in order to enhance the flow of your texts and structure ideas following an organizing principle. Next, the chapter considers 'micro structuring' at the paragraph level. At the end of the chapter you will find 'problem-shooting' checklists that deal with common grammar and English use problems such as sentence fragments, incorrect punctuation and dangling modifiers.

• Chapter 2: Exploring Academic Genres

Chapter 2 elaborates on the principles explored in the first chapter. It illustrates how these principles work for the typical texts or genres you will be asked to produce at the different levels of your undergraduate studies. In line with the demands of most university courses, the chapter works from description to argumentation. It thus starts with the generic academic essay and moves on to explore more specific genres such as the care critique and the article review. In the last part of the chapter, you will examine argumentation for the argumentative essay.

Chapter 3: Writing Processes in Academic Writing

This chapter will help you explore two complex writing processes: reflection and critical thinking. You will start by looking at what reflection involves and at how the different stages of the reflection cycle can be incorporated into the reflective essay. The chapter then introduces you to the principles of critical thinking and how you can use these principles to evaluate your sources of reference.

1 An Introduction to Academic Writing

At the end of this chapter, you should be able to:

- ▶ recognize the five basic principles of planning in academic writing
- ▶ identify the three elements in essay questions and follow marking criteria
- ▶ understand gathering, organizing and structuring information
- ▶ reproduce the generic structure of academic texts
- ▶ identify main problems with sentence fragments, cohesion, dangling modifiers and punctuation

● The basics of planning in academic writing

Have you ever written a letter? An email? Even a short mobile text? If you have, you wrote for a purpose. It was a **purposeful activity**. Academic writing is also a purposeful activity. When you write an assignment, you have a definite purpose in mind. You want a particular audience (who?) to have information (what?) with a specific focus (what exactly?). You have reasons for doing so (why?), and you are delivering the information in a certain way, such as describing, discussing or analysing (how?).

These question words (*who, what, what exactly, why* and *how*) can be your **guiding prompts** when you plan your next piece of writing.

Let us look at an example. Suppose you had to write an essay on the following: *Midwife means 'with woman'. Discuss how the midwife should care for the woman in the second stage of labour.* You could use the five question words above to ask yourself some guiding questions. For instance,

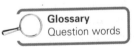

Glossary
Question words

Audience: **Who** am I writing the essay for? *Lecturer.*

Topic: **What** is the essay going to be about? *Midwife care for the woman in labour.*

Focus: **What exactly** am I going to focus on? *Some ways in which the midwife can provide care in the second stage of labour.*

Rationale: **Why** am I going to focus on some ways of providing care and not others? *They are the most crucial at this stage of labour.*

Signpost: **How** am I going to deliver the information? *By discussing the different ways the midwife can provide the care.*

These questions will help you choose the right information for your essay as well as the right amount of information for your audience. Your course lecturer, your audience in this case, already knows the answer to the essay question and probably expects you will answer it in a certain way. But your lecturer does not exactly know what information you will choose or why you will choose it. This is the **rationale** for your essay. It is what makes your essay unique – only you will choose to deal with the topic in the way you have decided.

These questions give you the five basic principles of essay planning. They will help you organize your ideas and structure your information so that your

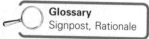

essay has the focus you want it to have. Organizing and structuring your information in this way will also improve the flow of your texts.
You will need more information to develop your essay, but the five questions give you the basic approach to planning any academic text. When your lecturer finishes reading your assignment, s/he should know why you have answered the essay question the way you have.

● Planning and structuring principles

Let us now examine one possible way of planning your essays according to the five basic questions that represent basic **planning and structuring principles**. Figure 1.1 shows how you can go about planning to answer an essay question. The figure illustrates how you can organize your essay (for example from general to specific) and how you can structure it (from background information to example). When you decide to arrange the information in your text from general to specific, as in this case, or from most to least important or chronologically (from most recent to oldest), you are using an **organization principle**. But, when you decide that your text will present

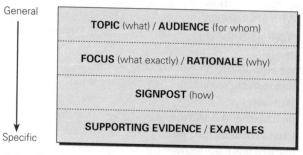

Figure 1.1   Planning essays

your reader with some background information before the focus and the rationale, as shown in Figure 1.1, you are planning the **structuring principle** for your text.

Remember that whereas organization can easily be changed, structure is not as flexible. Structure is connected with the way we transmit and understand new and given information. Structuring tends to be fairly fixed, and it largely depends on the language you are using. In English writing, background information normally precedes supporting examples. It is always a good idea to choose your organizing principle first and then decide on the most appropriate structure for your information.

You may decide, for example, that the information in your essay will be organized from general to specific. Then you may choose to structure it giving the background information first, and then the examples. Thus, your text will present,

- **background information** on the topic (what);
- the **focus** (what exactly);
- the **rationale** for answering the essay question in a particular way (why);
- the **signpost** (how the information will be delivered: by description, analysis, discussion, etc.).

Understanding essay questions

You will find many of the ideas we have just discussed in essay questions themselves. Essay questions can tell you what information to include (what), what aspects of that information to include (what exactly) and how you should deliver such aspects (how). If you analyse essay questions carefully, you will discover that most contain these three basic elements: the **topic**, the **focus** and the **signpost**. How you approach the topic is entirely up to you and, as we said, it is what makes your essay different from all other essays.

Let us consider again the essay question:

> *Midwife means 'with woman'. Discuss how the midwife should care for the woman in the second stage of labour.*

The topic is the care that the midwife should provide for the woman. This is very broad and you could include many things in your discussion. You could, for example, think of pre-natal and post-natal care, health promotion, care to meet the woman's social needs, and the like. However, the essay question asks about *the second stage of labour*. Many of these aspects of midwifery care are only *indirectly* connected to the second stage of labour which is the aspect on which you need to focus your writing. Therefore, you need to narrow down your focus. You should then consider things like:

- How does the midwife's role change in the second stage?
- How do the woman's needs change in the second stage?
- This stage is called the 'pushing stage'; what is actually happening?
- Should the midwife go for 'spontaneous pushing' or 'sustained directed bearing down efforts'?
- How can the midwife support the woman emotionally until the baby is born?

Narrowing down will help you stay focused and avoid including information that is not relevant to the topic. Finally, you should look at the verb to see how your lecturer expects you to develop your answer. The verb in the

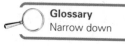

Glossary
Narrow down

question will indicate how you need to signpost your essay. What is the verb in the example essay question? Does it ask you to,

- say what is right or wrong about the care that the midwife should provide in the second stage of labour?
- examine different aspects of the care in the second stage of labour?

'Discuss' does not mean to say what is right or wrong. It means to examine different aspects of a topic. You could, for instance, think of the midwife care in terms of physical support (for example suggesting alternative positions for women without epidural anaesthesia, helping with contractions) and of emotional support (for example dealing with intense emotions and sensations). In this way, you could examine the different roles that the midwife could play in the second stage and, using **supporting evidence** from the literature (see later in the chapter), discuss alternatives in relation to physical and emotional support. As this example shows, verbs in essay

Glossary
Supporting evidence

questions are essential to understand how you are supposed to signpost your essay.

Let us look at another example. This time we will examine a typical question for nursing students:

Evaluate the importance of effective communication in nursing.

Activity 1.1

The table below lists the verbs you will see most often used in essay questions. Write the meaning of each verb in your own words. You do not need to provide complete sentences; key words will do. Use a dictionary if you are not sure of the meanings. 'Argue' and 'discuss' have been done for you as examples.

Verb	Definition	Additional information
Analyse		
Argue	To give reasons why something is right or wrong, true or untrue.	To persuade people.
Classify		
Demonstrate		
Differentiate		
Discuss	To examine in detail, showing the different opinions or ideas about something.	Frequently confused with 'argue', but a more balanced response is required in 'discuss'.
Evaluate		
Examine		
Explain		
Identify		
Outline		
Produce		

Answers See suggested answers on page 188

Again, you should identify the topic first: *communication in nursing*. Remember that topics tend to be broad. So you will need a focus. In this example question, the focus is given by the phrase 'the importance of effective communication'. You will need to tell your reader what 'effective communication in nursing' is and 'why it is important'.

You could, for example, include ideas such as 'communication with other nurses, clients, and the client's family', 'what makes each type of communication effective', 'the importance of verbal communication on admission to hospital', and the like.

Finally, you need to consider the signpost; that is, the action you are asked to take in relation to the topic and its focus. In this example, the action is 'evaluate', so you are to judge the value of effective communication in nursing to form an opinion about it (see Activity 1.1 above and the suggested answers at the back of the book).

● Interpreting and using marking criteria

As well as the essay question, you should also look at the **marking criteria** for the essay. These criteria are an important source of information for you. They will help you make decisions on what to include in your essay. Using

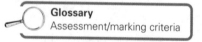

Glossary
Assessment/marking criteria

the marking criteria at the planning stage will improve your chances of getting a higher mark.

Here is another example. This is a question for a 1,000 word reflective essay and its accompanying marking criteria:

Discuss how your transferable skills of communication, effective learning, teamwork, numeracy and personal and career development have developed during the semester.

Criteria	Comments
1 Work neatly presented and easy to read	
2 Evidence of self-assessment of skills at beginning of semester	
3 Balanced view of the progress made in each of the skills	
4 Identification of further developmental needs	
5 Correct spelling and grammar	
6 List of references included	

Table 1.1   Sample marking criteria for a short essay

Did you realize that half the total marking criteria for this assignment are for the conventions of academic writing? Let us examine each of these three criteria in more detail.

Criterion 1 refers to the presentation of your work and how easy it is to read. A well-presented essay may get a higher mark than a disorganized and poorly presented one. Here are some important things to keep in mind. Your essay should be:

- word processed, with no typing errors;
- double-spaced throughout;
- written in a legible **font style** and **font size** – normally using Times New Roman or Arial, 11 or 12 pt;
- presented with generous margins – generally 2 to 2.5 centimetres all around;

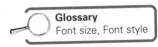

Glossary
Font size, Font style

- correctly introduced (see the section on paragraphing below);
- adequately paragraphed (ditto).

Criterion 5 is also connected with how easy your essay is to read. If the spelling and grammar are correct, you will improve your chances of getting a better mark. You should:

- use the word processor spell-check, though it is always safer to use a dictionary;
- refer to grammar guides if you are unsure of correct uses of the language (see the section on grammar and English use below, and Further Readings and Resources at the end of the book).

Criterion 6 is about referencing, which is discussed in Chapter 10, although here are some basic considerations connected with references. When you prepare your **list of references**, you have to remember to:

- include only those references you have mentioned in the body of your text;

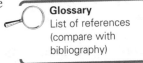

Glossary
List of references
(compare with
bibliography)

- organize the list of references alphabetically;
- include the basic information about the references;
- make sure there is no discrepancy between the references on the list and those in the text.

Now that you have

- examined the essay question, and
- analysed the marking criteria,

you are ready to start the final stage in planning: searching for the information that you will include in your essay.

Gathering information

This final stage in planning is known as 'search and select'. This simply means that you collect lots of information, then you choose the most useful. These two processes are closely linked, and are important for organizing and structuring information before you start writing your essay. Figure 1.2 illustrates the links between them.

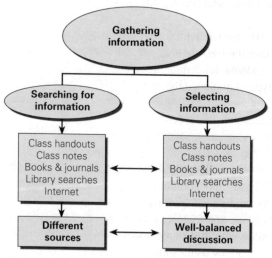

Figure 1.2   The process of gathering information

Searching for information

Where can you start searching for information? Class handouts and class notes can provide an excellent starting point, they may contain references which have been suggested by lecturers, normally in a recommended reading list. These sources of 'pre-selected information' can help you reduce the anxiety created by having to look at too many sources.

The internet is another source of information, but it can also be a source of confusion. When you do an internet search, remember to use key words instead of phrases. For instance, if you wanted to do a search for

> *Midwife means 'with woman'. Discuss how the midwife should care for the woman in the second stage of labour.*

you would be better off using key words like 'second stage of labour'. This will reduce the number of hits you will get back as a response to your search. Alternatively, if you want to search for the whole phrase 'the second stage of labour', use inverted commas at the beginning and end of the phase so as to avoid hitting pages containing meaningless words such as 'the' and 'of'.

A second word of warning about the internet relates to the quality of information you may find. Unlike other sources (such as journals and books), the contents of websites may not be safeguarded for their accuracy and correctness. There are no 'editorial boards' to make sure that what gets published is accurate and correct. Always check for things such as:

- who is responsible for the website;
- whether the website is associated with or recognized by a council;
- the academic credential of the person writing the information;
- the type of audience the website was designed for.

Once you have established a relationship of trust with a given website, then you can use its information safely.

A more reliable source of information for your academic activities is databases. Access to online databases will be provided by your university library. Academic databases may contain information about books, journals, newspapers, reports, and so on. You have to keep in mind that each source is different in its scope and features so it is always a good idea to start by first becoming familiar with the source you will be using. The two main ways to search databases are by using subject headings, also called 'descriptors', and keywords. You can get more detailed information on how to use the databases available at your university by using the 'Help' function in the database or by asking a librarian at your university library.

Selecting information

Not all the sources of information you have chosen will find a home in your essay. You will still have to **select** the most appropriate pieces. As shown in Figure 1.2, there are various principles you can follow. You can select information by:

- its topic;
- its focus;
- how closely connected it is to your focus;
- its quality;
- whether it is *evidence-based*.

It is also important that you present your reader with an objective and balanced account. For this, you will need to include not only those sources of information that confirm your position but also those that challenge it. We will return to this point when we deal with argumentation in Chapter 2 and, especially, in Chapter 6.

If you manage to strike a balance between these types of sources (books, journal articles and internet sources), you will provide your readers with **different sources** of good quality and updated information. Lecturers will want to see this in your assignments.

If you manage to consider not only relevant and **evidence-based** argu-

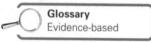
Glossary
Evidence-based

ments that support the points you want to make but also those that challenge your arguments, you will provide your audience with a **well-balanced discussion**. Lecturers will want to see this in your assignments too!

● Organizing and structuring information

Now it is time to decide how you will **organize and structure** your essay. Remember that organizing and structuring are two related, but slightly different processes. Organization has to do with order, while structuring refers to patterns. If you were working on the different ways the midwife can support the woman in the second stage of labour, how could you organize these ways?

One way is by listing. When you list aspects, or ways like in this case, you isolate them and thus you can identify them more clearly. There is also an element of 'classifying' here. Classifying helps with logical thinking, achieving balance and clearer writing. Do not worry about the order of the elements in your list; you can change the order later on. Use bullets rather than numbers so you do not get any particular order fixed in your head at this stage.

For example, you can list the ways in which the midwife can support the woman physically and emotionally:

Supporting women in the second stage of labour

A *Physical support*
- Monitor the fetal heart
- Assess and protect the perineum
- Provide equipment e.g. beanbag

B *Emotional support*
- Talk her through the process
- Encourage verbally
- Support choice of position

The next step is to give the selected items a certain order. This step should always be guided by some principle. As we discussed above, you can organize them chronologically, in order of importance, or by dealing with the most difficult first. In this case we will organize the items following a chronological order:

Supporting women in the second stage of labour

1 *Physical support*
1.1 Monitor the fetal heart
1.2 Provide equipment e.g. beanbag
1.3 Assess and protect the perineum

2 *Emotional support*
2.1 Support choice of position
2.2 Encourage verbally
2.3 Talk her through the process

Notice that you can now change bullets into numbers as this is the order in which the essay will be developed.

Activity 1.2

Here are some scrambled ideas about the second essay question we considered above: *Evaluate the importance of effective communication in nursing.* How would you organise and structure them to write an essay on this question? You may need to leave some out, depending on the rationale you have chosen.

The importance of effective communication in nursing

- Collaboration and negotiation skills with clients and families
- Common barriers to effective communication
- Communication as a therapeutic space
- Communicating with the family
- Work teams in nursing practice
- Dealing with aggression
- Focusing on feelings, being warm and non-judgemental
- Self-disclosure and small groups
- Facilitating empathy

Answers See suggested answers on page 189.

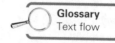

Glossary
Text flow

Organizing and structuring will help the ideas in your **text flow** more smoothly, while enhancing your chances of a higher mark.

Paragraphing information

Now that you have finished planning, it is time to shape your information into texts. This process is called '**paragraphing**'. Paragraphing refers to putting information into 'blocks' or paragraphs which contain one principal idea.

Activity 1.3

Read the following paragraph and answer the questions below.

Nurses can work in many healthcare settings, which gives them the opportunity to gain experience in all aspects of caring for clients and their families. Nurses can thus build their professional career in many different ways. They may choose to become clinical specialists or consultant nurses, or they can opt for managerial positions as a head of nursing services or supervisor of other nurses. Some may prefer to pursue an academic career in education and research. These are just a few examples of the opportunities that nurses currently have to develop their professional interests.

The paragraph has five sentences. Can you identify,

1   the sentence that introduces the general idea of the text (**topic**)?

2   another sentence that provides the focus/point of view of the topic (**focus**)?

3   the examples that develop/support the focus (**examples/evidence**)?

4   the sentence that brings the text to an end (**conclusion**)?

Answers See suggested answers on page 190.

The first sentence in a paragraph sets the scene for the reader. It discloses the **topic** of the text; that is why it is usually called the 'topic sentence'. This sentence provides the reader with enough background information to understand the text.

The topic and the focus in the paragraph above tell us that nurses can build a professional career in many different ways. But what are these ways? To answer this question, we need to go on reading and find either **examples** or **evidence** that support the claims made in the focus. The text above uses examples to do this. After the text presents examples exploring different possibilities for nurses, it moves on to a conclusion. The **conclusion**, the fifth sentence in the example, brings a text to an end in a satisfactory manner.

But what is a *satisfactory manner*? The answer is in the focus of your text. When you present your readers with the focus of your text, you create certain expectations in them. For example, if you said you would discuss 'the three fundamental reasons that make the third stage of labour the most critical', your reader would immediately expect to read three fundamental reasons why you consider the third stage of labour the most critical.

Also a satisfactory conclusion takes the reader back to the focus of the text. In the text about careers for nurses, we can clearly see how the conclusion **rephrases** (states the same idea by using similar words) the focus of the text. Thus, we can draw a parallel between the focus of the text ('nurses can thus build their professional career in many different ways') and its conclusion ('these are just few examples of the opportunities that nurses have to develop their professional interests.'). This conclusion is also satisfactory because it gives the reader

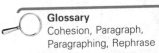

Glossary
Cohesion, Paragraph,
Paragraphing, Rephrase

something further to think about. The writer is inviting the reader to 'engage' with the ideas in the text by thinking of other ways that nurses can develop their careers or professional interests. Good conclusions always leave the reader with something to think about.

There is one last thing we need to consider: how all these parts of the text have been put together. This is called '**cohesion**'. Cohesion is the 'glue' that sticks the text together. You can create cohesion by:

- repeating key words that remind the reader of what the text is about and link the ideas expressed in different sentences;
- using a network of words (e.g. nurses, nursing, care, clients, etc.) that helps the writer put ideas together, while avoiding heavy repetition of the same word or words;
- using connectives (e.g. and, but, thus) that give unity to the text and show the connection between one idea and the next, one sentence and the next or even one text and the next (see the section on grammar and English use below).

● From paragraph to essay

The basic structure we have just analysed is sometimes referred to as the generic structure of a paragraph. A generic structure is like the 'backbone' of a text that can be used to generate similar texts. You can use this generic structure again and again every time you need to create a new paragraph.

The generic structure of a paragraph can be expanded to create the generic structure of an essay, and Figure 1.3 shows how the generic structure of a short text like the paragraph about careers for nurses can be expanded to create the structure of an essay.

The inverted triangle in the essay introduction represents the general-to-specific way in which information has been organized. In the conclusion, on the other hand, information has been organized from specific to general. We will come back to this at the end of this section.

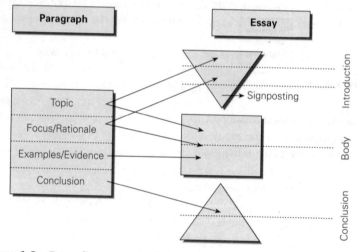

Figure 1.3   Expanding a paragraph into an essay

Sources: Adapted from Oshima and Hogue (1998), and Swales and Feak (1994).

The function of each part of a paragraph (for example the topic sentence provides the reader with background information about the text) can be mirrored in the function of each part of an essay. So, the introduction of an essay will first present the topic, then the focus, and then the rationale. The only function that we do not frequently find in a paragraph but which should be present in the introduction of an essay is signposting (how you will deliver the information in your essay).

Let us look (Figure 1.4) at how the topic and the focus in the paragraph about careers for nurses can be expanded into the introduction of a short essay.

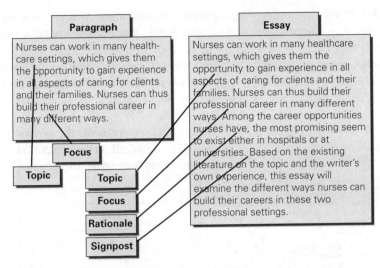

Figure 1.4   From paragraph to essay – example 1

The examples used to support the claims we have made in the focus of the paragraph and in the essay introduction can be organized in different paragraphs in the body of the essay. Figure 1.5 illustrates one way of doing this.

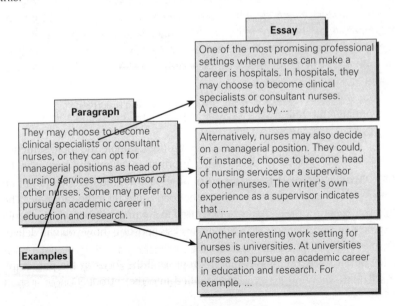

Figure 1.5   From paragraph to essay – example 2

Notice how each supporting example has generated one body paragraph in the essay. Can you also see how each of the paragraphs in the body of the essay follows the generic structure we discussed above: topic, focus and evidence or examples to support the claims? Figure 1.6 now shows how the conclusion in the paragraph about careers for nurses can be expanded into the concluding paragraph of the essay.

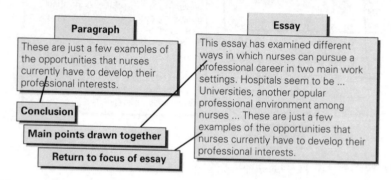

Figure 1.6   From paragraph to essay – example 3

As you can see, the concluding paragraph in the essay first draws together the main points mentioned in the body by summarizing them. It then returns to the focus of the essay. Notice also that while the information in the introductory paragraph is organized from general to specific, the organization of the information in the conclusion goes from specific to general. Although you may come across variations of this kind of essay organization and structuring, this is a typical ordering and patterning of information in an academic essay.

You will find more on planning, organizing and structuring specific assignments (the reflective essay, the care critique and the like) in Part 2 of the book.

● Grammar and English use

This last section of the chapter deals with some of the main grammar and language-use problems that many students experience when writing academically. We look at sentence fragments, cohesion, dangling modifiers and punctuation. For easy referencing, these problems are examined in the form of a trouble-shooting list. If you feel you need more detail on any of these topics, see the Glossary of Key Terms and the list of Further Readings and Resources at the end of the book.

Sentence fragments

Sentence fragments are incomplete pieces of writing which do not make sense on their own. The most common fragments are:

- phrases without a main verb (e.g. *All treatments available at hospitals.*);
- parts of a longer sentence which have been used independently (e.g. *Because they made the wrong decision.*);
- phrases with a verb but without a subject (e.g. *In the end decided to go for a caesarean operation.*).

Problem	Solution
Phrase without a main verb Some more comments about the procedures. (a phrase)	**Add a verb** Some more comments were made about the procedures.
Unconnected fragment Patients were asked to sign consent forms. Before the doctors made a final decision. (a part of the previous sentence)	**Join the two parts to make one sentence** Patients were asked to sign consent forms before the doctors made a final decision.
Missing subject Through not carefully monitoring the fetus created a risky situation for both the mother and the baby. (no subject)	**Add the doer of the action** Through not carefully monitoring the fetus, they created a risky situation for both the mother and the baby.

Table 1.2   Sentence fragments

Cohesion

Cohesion refers to the use of words or phrases that allow you to put parts of a text together. You can provide cohesion by, for example, repeating key words, creating a network of similar words, and using connectives (words or phrases that connect, e.g. and, but, so). Cohesion is important to make sure the text flows and to link ideas, paragraphs and longer texts.

Problem	Solution
Group of choppy sentences Nurses can specialize in different areas. They can, for example, choose to do mental health, dual diagnosis. They can also choose neonatal nursing. Nurses can specialize within hospitals. They can work as a school nurse. They can move out into the community.	**Use connectives** Nurses can specialize in different areas. They can, for example, choose to do mental health, dual diagnosis *or* neonatal nursing. They can also specialize within hospitals, work as a school nurse or move out into the community.
Little cohesion Breastfeeding can help the mother have a faster recovery after childbirth. The hormones that are normally released during nursing help the uterus return to its normal size. It can reduce bleeding. Nursing mothers can lose weight more easily.	**Use a connective** Breastfeeding can help the mother have a faster recovery after child birth. The hormones that are normally released during nursing help the uterus return to its normal size. It can *also* reduce bleeding. *In addition*, it has been found that nursing mothers can lose weight more easily.
Very little cohesion Nurses can work in many health care settings, which gives them the opportunity to gain experience in all aspects of care. They can thus build their career in many different ways.	**Create a network of words** *Nurses* can work in many healthcare settings, which gives them the opportunity to gain experience in all aspects of care for *clients* and their *families*. *Nurses* can thus build their *professional* career in many different ways.

Table 1.3   Sentence cohesion

Dangling modifiers

A dangling modifier is a word or a phrase that has no clear connection with the rest of the sentence. For example:

> *Having asked all patients for their consent, the survey was carried out.*

In this case, 'having asked all patients for their consent' is dangling (loosely or not clearly connected with the following part of the sentence). One important point to remember here is that phrases at the beginning of a sentence do not have a stated subject but take the subject of the following sentence, sometimes creating a humorous effect. Consider another example which appeared in an American newspaper article:

> *While driving on Greenwood Avenue yesterday afternoon, a tree began to fall toward Wendy H's car. (As is, it sounds as if the tree was driving!)*

Problem	Solution
Dangling modifier Having finished the shift, all uniforms worn on the day were sent to the laundry.	**Change the subject of the sentence** Having finished the shift, *the caretakers* sent all uniforms worn on the day to the laundry. **or** **Add a subject to the first part** When *the shift* was finished, all uniforms worn on the day were sent to the laundry.
Dangling modifier Without numeracy skills, drugs cannot be administered to patients.	**Change the subject of the sentence** Without numeracy skills, *nurses* cannot administer drugs to patients. **or** **Add a subject to the first part** If nurses do not have numeracy skills, they cannot administer drugs to their patients.

Table 1.4   Dangling modifiers

Punctuation

Punctuation is used to signal pause, emphasis, expansion or clarification. The most frequently used punctuation marks are the *colon, comma, dash, full stop, parentheses, quotation marks* and *semicolon*.

> **Glossary**
> Punctuation marks

Problem	Solution
At this hospital, nurses can specialize in one of three areas, mental health, dual diagnosis or neonatal nursing.	**Use a colon to introduce other related ideas** At this hospital, nurses can specialize in one of three areas: mental health, dual diagnosis or neonatal nursing. **NB**: if the colon introduces a list of objects, names, or phrases, they should be separated by commas. If the colon introduces complete sentences, they should be separated by semi-colons (;).
Before they can register with the council nurses have to have the necessary qualifications.	**Add a comma after an introductory sentence** Before they can register with the council, nurses have to have the necessary qualifications.
After finishing their shift all midwives should sign the register.	**Add a comma after an introductory phrase** After finishing their shift, all midwives should sign the register.
The results contradicted previous studies. However replication of this study has been highly recommended.	**Add a comma after an introductory connective** The results contradicted previous studies. However, replication of this study has been highly recommended.
Doctors, nurses and consultants, considered all the possible ways of saving his life.	**Delete the comma that separates the subject** (what is being talked about) **from the verb** Doctors, nurses and consultants considered all the possible ways of saving his life.

Problem	Solution
Organization, structuring and paragraphing, such are the qualities of good academic writing.	**Mark off a summarizing statement with a dash** Organization, structuring and paragraphing – such are the qualities of good academic writing.
The midwife should provide her clients with all the necessary information for them to make informed decisions	**Finish a complete sentence** (not a question or exclamation) **with a full stop** The midwife should provide her clients with all the necessary information for them to make informed decisions.
The consultant, who had received more than one prize, someone said more than a dozen, denied the accusation.	**Put extra, non-essential, information between parentheses** The consultant, who had received more than one prize (someone said more than a dozen), denied the accusation.
When this happens, health promotion has proven to be the most effective strategy (Stallen, 2003).	**Use quotation marks to enclose somebody else's words** When this happens, health promotion 'has proven to be the most effective strategy' (Stallen, 2003, p. 345). Also see Chapters 9 and 10.
They tried all possible ways to save his life however, his heart did not restart.	**Use a semicolon before a connective that connects two sentences** They tried all possible ways to save his life; however, his heart did not restart.

Table 1.5   Problems with punctuation

Revising the objectives of this chapter

Tick those objectives you feel you have achieved and review those you have not yet managed to accomplish. Then, complete the **Achievement Chart** at the back of the book.

In this chapter, you have learnt to:

☐ recognize the five basic principles of planning in academic writing

☐ identify the three elements in essay questions and follow marking criteria

☐ understand gathering, organizing and structuring information

☐ reproduce the generic structure of academic texts

☐ identify main problems with sentence fragments, cohesion, dangling modifiers and punctuation

2 Exploring Academic Genres

At the end of this chapter, you should be able to:

- ▶ recognize the difference between description and argumentation
- ▶ identify the main academic genres in nursing and midwifery
- ▶ understand the purpose and the structure of these genres
- ▶ identify main language items used in descriptive and critical writing

● From description to argumentation

Have you noticed that an ad for a 'room to let', for example, has a different function from a letter to the editor of a newspaper? Compare these two samples:

Sir,
I was really surprised to read that the association of clinical diabetologists claims that more consultants are needed to cope with the increasing epidemic when they know too well that most diabetes care lies in the hands of the GP.
    What we REALLY need is more staff and facilities to help GP practices manage the increasing number of patients suffering from diabetes.
    Have they not heard that many hospital diabetologists insist on keeping diabetes care in the community?

Dr. D. T.
London

— ROOM TO LET —
A double room with a fridge, new double bed, newly furnished, with a three-door wardrobe, drawer unit and bedside table. TV with cable and internet facility ready. Two large windows. 2 minutes from tube station.

Figure 2.1   'Room to let' vs 'letter to the editor'

While the ad for the room describes its size, furniture, location, etc., the letter to the editor presents a particular claim about a topic recently discussed in the newspaper. The ad is descriptive; the letter to the editor is argumentative.

As an undergraduate student of nursing or midwifery, you will be asked to produce both descriptive and argumentative writing. In the first year of your programme, you will be required to write some descriptive essays, in which you mostly describe facts, sometimes with a small amount of analysis. This is normally referred to as 'level-1 writing' and is broadly equivalent to Certificate (C) level in the Quality Assurance Agency (QAA) Framework for Higher Education Qualifications in England, Wales and Northern Ireland.

Towards the end of the first year and beginning of the second, you will need to start developing your higher level cognitive skills. This is when you start writing more evaluative **genres** such as the **care critique** and the **article review**. In the final year of your programme, you will have to write **argumentative essays**, showing a **critical analysis** of the issues explored.

This progression from description to argumentation can be charted on a cline. This cline, shown in Figure 2.2, illustrates how description, critical skills and argumentation are combined as you progress on your programme of study.

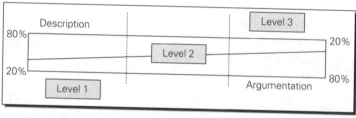

Figure 2.2 The description-argumentation cline

Glossary
Genres, Argumentative writing, Care critique, Article review, Critical analysis

No piece of writing can be 100% descriptive or 100% argumentative. It will always be a combination of the two, but the percentage of each changes as your writing becomes more complex. Figure 2.2 shows how descriptive and argumentative skills combine along the cline. Although there are no hard and fast rules for hitting the winning formula, it is fairly common to find an 80–20 combination (80% description and 20% analysis) at the descriptive end of the cline.

Nearing the end of the first year, this combination already starts to change. Around your second year of study, the genres you will be asked to write require a 40–60 combination, weighting the formula in favour of argumentation. This is called 'writing at level 2' and is roughly equivalent to Intermediate (I) level in the QAA Framework. Towards the completion of your programme, the combination of description and argumentation is completely reversed. At this other end of the cline, you will be producing argumentative essays which require a combination of 20% description and 80% argumentation. This is 'level-3 writing' and should lead to the achievement of some of the Honours (H) level learning outcomes in the QAA Framework.

The genres you will be required to write can be structurally based on a generic essay which we call the *academic essay*. This is what we will discuss in the next section.

● The academic essay

The academic essay is also known as the three-section essay. It normally has an introductory section, a main body and a concluding section. The way information is organized and structured in this essay is similar to the way the essay about careers for nurses in Chapter 1 was organized.

The academic essay is a **generic genre** that can be used for many purposes. It may:

- describe facts, issues, etc. (the descriptive essay);
- identify logical relationships (the explanatory essay); or
- compare two or more issues or aspects of a topic (the comparative essay).

It is important to remember that the purpose of your essay should reflect the purpose of the essay question, mainly given by its verb. Is your essay supposed to *describe*, *explain*, *compare* or *discuss*? You should also keep in mind that the functions of each section (introduction, body and conclusion) should agree with the general function of your essay. This will enhance the structure and the flow of your text.

> **Glossary**
> Generic genre

In this section of the chapter we will discuss the function of each of the parts of the academic essay, but we will focus mainly on the introduction, as it is here where you signal what the essay will do: describe, explain, identify, compare, and so on.

The introduction
One function of the introduction is to tell your reader how you plan to develop your essay (see also Chapter 1). There are several ways in which you may do this, based on what the essay question asks you to do. You may, for example, need to describe facts, identify **logical relationships** or compare issues of a topic.

It is important that you can identify the connection between your purpose for writing (to answer the question) and the type of essay you need to write

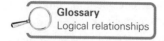

Glossary
Logical relationships

(to follow the verb in the question). If the essay question requires you to write an article review, for example, then your response to the question will have to evaluate the merits of such a piece of writing. You will then need to produce an evaluative essay and you will signpost your introduction using verbs such as 'evaluate', 'judge' and 'analyse', which will at the same time reflect the verb in the question (see the section on grammar and English use later in the chapter). These considerations will help you choose the best type of essay to answer the questions you were given.

Remember that signposting the introduction will create certain expectations in your reader's mind, and it is your responsibility as a writer to make sure that these expectations are met in the rest of your essay. If, for example, you signpost your essay with,

> *This essay will examine the value of vaginal examination of pregnant women on hospital admission*

what expectations will your reader have? You have signposted an evaluation. You have told your reader that you will 'examine the value of something'. They will expect you to evaluate the worth of doing vaginal examinations when a pregnant woman is admitted to hospital. They will expect you to use words such as 'analyse' and 'examine'. They will not expect a description of how vaginal examinations are carried out on admission to hospital, for example. If you give such a description, your reader will be disappointed, because you failed to meet the expectations you created in their mind.

Similarly, if your introduction states that 'The essay will present a description of the latest medical technologies for the ICU' but your readers find a debate on ethical problems instead, they will feel dissatisfied. They were expecting to find a description, not a debate. Make sure your essay has achieved what its introduction promised. Reader disappointment usually results from unmet expectations. And disappointment of this sort will translate into a low mark for you.

The other important function of the introduction is to outline the content of the essay. The content of your essay is partly announced in the topic sentence, but mainly in the focus (see Chapter 1). However, it is always a good idea to wait until you have planned the body of your essay to outline the content in the introduction.

As you can see, the value of the introduction cannot be underestimated. The introduction will help you keep focused and organized. It will also serve as the map of the territory for the reader. It will show the readers the path you have planned for them, and what content they can expect to find in the body.

The main body

What should the paragraphs in the body of an academic essay do? They should develop the focus and the rationale that you presented your reader with in the introduction. You will mainly accomplish this by presenting your supporting evidence in blocks of information (see also Chapter 1). Each of these blocks will deal with one issue as you signposted it in your introduction, and may require one or several paragraphs to do so.

Let us take the example about vaginal examinations. You may want to assess their value as (a) a method of measuring progress in labour, and (b) a method of assessing abnormal presentations of the foetus. Then your reader may expect two fairly long body sections, each dealing with one of these. This is shown in Figure 2.3.

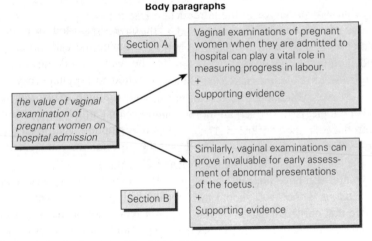

Body paragraphs

Section A

Vaginal examinations of pregnant women when they are admitted to hospital can play a vital role in measuring progress in labour.
+
Supporting evidence

the value of vaginal examination of pregnant women on hospital admission

Similarly, vaginal examinations can prove invaluable for early assessment of abnormal presentations of the foetus.
+
Supporting evidence

Section B

Figure 2.3   Body paragraphs in an essay

Let us look at another example of how to structure information in the body of an academic essay. Your introduction indicated *'This essay will describe the latest medical technologies for the ICU'*. It will focus particularly on three of the most important – electronic charting, boom technology and dispensing systems. The body of your essay would then need one block for each of these technologies. For example, it could include one or more paragraphs on each of following:

- electronic charting on nurses' stations;

- boom technology;
- automated dispensing systems for pharmaceuticals.

In each of these blocks, you could support your claims by describing, but not arguing for or against, the main features of these technologies. You would need to describe what these technologies are and how they function, including enough information to cover them adequately. In this way, you will provide your reader with a fairly complete picture of the technological advances for critical care, while meeting the expectations you created in them.

The conclusion

What does the conclusion do? It summarizes or rounds off the main issues that you announced in the introduction and explored in the body of the essay. Apart from bringing together the issues presented in the body, the conclusion will normally draw the reader's attention back to the focus of the essay that was presented in the introduction (see also Chapter 1). This will create a sense of satisfaction in the reader. The expectations your introduction creates in their mind are later met in the body of your essay, and finally rounded off in the conclusion.

Conclusions sometimes leave the reader with something to think about as well. However, you should be careful not to confuse this with new issues about the topic. Issues which are not announced in the introduction cannot be introduced in the conclusion. The conclusion is the part where you 'close doors' rather than open them.

Table 2.1 on page 32 presents a checklist of things you may need to review after you have finished writing your essays. If your answer to any of the questions is 'no', you should then decide what action you will take to improve that particular aspect of your essay. As you use the checklist more regularly, add new questions to it so that it becomes more relevant to your needs as a writer.

The academic essay may serve as the basis upon which other genres can be planned and structured. You will probably have to make some adaptations to the basic structure. For example, in a longer essay you will have more paragraphs or more references to adequately develop and support your information. However, even longer essays will still show the basic structural elements: introduction, body and conclusion. The rest of the chapter explores longer genres such as the care critique, the review article and the argumentative essay.

Activity 2.1

Here are three essay questions and the introductions that have been written to answer them. As you read the introductions, try and evaluate how effective they are. Think of some reasons to back up your decisions. You may use these questions to guide you:

- Can you identify the **topic**, **focus** and **signpost** of the essay?
- Do they provide the reader with **enough information** to know what the text will be about?
- Can you say what you **expect to find** in the body of each of the essays?

What does providing care for the critically ill patient involve? Discuss.

Introduction 1
Despite the great advances in medical treatments, many patients spend their final hours in intensive care units (ICU). More often than not, people are afraid of having a high-technology death with prolonged periods of suffering, and taxing obligations for their family. Caring for the critically ill patient in an intensive care unit then means that difficult ethical problems must be faced and resolved.

Analyse the role of reassurance in nursing care.

Introduction 2
There are various roles that a nurse is supposed to carry out, and among the different personal qualities that these roles involve reassurance seems to be the most important one. Reassurance has been described as a powerful element to ease patients' fears, concerns and anxieties during their stay in hospitals. This essay will explore the concept of reassurance in connection with the patient's concerns and anxieties when hospitalised. It will first discuss some definitions of reassurance in an attempt to isolate its main attributes.

Evaluate the value of models for treating dual diagnosis clients.

Introduction 3
Dual diagnosis specialists are becoming increasingly aware of the need to develop a treatment model that addresses the challenges posed by clients with severe mental health problems and a history of misuse of substances. There are a few intervention programmes to treat clients with a dual diagnosis. However, they are relatively new and have not been objectively evaluated for their effectiveness. In some countries, increasing attention to these issues is being paid and, as a result, several integrated approach treatment programmes have been set up. These involve specialised multidisciplinary teams, working to address the unmet needs of clients. This essay will briefly describe the existing models, and thoroughly examine their value. Against this background, the essay will evaluate the potentials of the new programmes in the light of the results obtained in their implementation.

Answers See suggested answers on page 190.

Questions	Yes/No	Action if 'no'
1 Have you chosen the best **type of essay** to answer the **essay question**?		
2 Have you presented the **introduction** clearly, indicating **topic** and **focus**?		
3 Have you signposted your **purpose** clearly (describe, explain, compare, etc.)?		
4 Have you **structured** the body of your essay **effectively** (e.g. one main idea developed in each paragraph)?		
5 Have you **written enough** about the subject to cover the focus adequately?		
6 Have you supported your main ideas by **specific examples** or **evidence**?		
7 Have you included only **information** that is **relevant** to the topic and the focus?		
8 Have you included **enough details** in your supporting information?		
9 Have you concluded in a **logical** and **satisfactory** manner?		

Table 2.1   Checklist for the academic essay

● The care critique: an introduction

This section of the chapter presents an introduction to the care critique, one of the most frequent genres in nursing and midwifery. Because it is so important, we'll take a closer look at it in Chapter 5.

Two terms normally associated with the care critique are 'criticize' and 'critique'. How do they compare?

- 'criticize' is related to the bad qualities of something and to showing disapproval. It is normally based on what the speaker or writer dislikes or thinks is wrong or inappropriate.
- 'critique', on the other hand, is associated with the writer's reaction to the value of something. 'To critique' means to present a balanced evaluation (what is good and bad) of what is being considered and 'a critique' is the essay you write when you do this.

Whereas criticism points out negative aspects, critiques analyse the value of something. The critique focuses on the object being analysed, rather than on the writer's subjective opinion or personal experience. In the care critique, the writer's focus of attention is the care, how effective, relevant and appropriate this care has proven to be, and the recommendations that he/she can make to improve the care provided.

The structure of the care critique will then show:

- an introduction, stating topic, focus and signpost;
- a body, identifying main issues in connection with topic and clinical practice;
- a conclusion, summarizing main issues and showing their link with focus; and
- recommendation/s (how care could be improved).

● The journal article review

The journal article review is a critical account of a published article. It critiques the main aspects and the contribution the article makes to knowledge. In nursing studies, articles used for review have normally been published in journals such as the *Critical Care Nurse*, the *Journal of the American Academy of Nurse Practitioners*, the *Journal of Nurse-Midwifery*, *Nurse Education Today*, and the *Journal of Advanced Nursing*.

The article review is normally between 3–4 pages long (between 800–1,000 words) and it is a piece of academic writing. This means you should observe conventions of style, organization and presentation (see also Chapter 1), as well as referencing conventions (see also Chapter 10).

Although you will need some kind of description and, for this, you will use descriptive language, the focus of your review should be on analysis and

Activity 2.2

Read the essay question and the marking criteria. Then, look at the outline for the care critique. Judging from the outline, how effective would you say the critique will be? Use the ratings provided below and be prepared to give reasons for your choice.

1: Very effective **2**: Effective **3**: Not very effective **4**: Not at all effective

Essay question: The role of the midwife in supporting a woman who chooses to smoke during pregnancy

Essay type: 3,000 word care critique

Marking criteria:
1 Work neatly presented, easy to read and within the word limit
2 Clear identification of issues relating to care
3 Able to articulate theory and practice
4 Knowledge of basic concepts and issues
5 Accurate and appropriate referencing

Outline:
Intro: Smoking during pregnancy, smoking cessation, statistics
Midwife plays a fundamental role (inform, support, help to make informed decisions, provide alternatives)
Care provided by an experienced midwife the writer observed
Essay will discuss support offered in terms of information and empowerment of the client

Body:
1   Present information about care provided
2   Identify issues (client's own choice, consequences for foetus, consequences for client, etc.)
3   Information:
how it was provided (explanation, materials, literature, etc)
what the midwife did with it
how the midwife checked information was understood and processed by client
4   Empowerment:
how information was used
how it helped client make informed decisions
the results
5   Analysis:
what was achieved by midwife's intervention
what could also have been done
what was ineffective and why

Conclusion: summarise main issues, draw attention to focus
Make recommendations: how support could be improved

Answers See suggested answers on page 191.

evaluation. In an article review, you are expected to do more than describe the contents of the article. You must also analyse and evaluate the methodology and findings of the research.

Your review should show that you can:

- think clearly and with originality;
- think critically;
- write concisely;
- write academically.

There are four essential steps in preparing to write an article review, as listed in Table 2.2.

	Steps	Comments
1	Draw up a list of questions to keep in mind while reading.	For instance, 'Who wrote the article?', 'What are their credentials?', 'When was it published?', 'Where was it published?', 'Do its contents seem to be well researched?'
2	Read the article more than once.	It's important that you become familiar with the article you're about to review. Read it for general understanding first, and then read it again (and again if necessary) for its content, methodology, and findings.
3	Read and take notes.	As you read the article for the second (or third) time, jot down things you notice or that attract your attention (e.g. inconsistencies). You will need these notes for outlining your review. Remember your review should *critique*, not only *describe* the article.
4	Read and network.	As you read it for the last time, try to make connections between the ideas or issues in this article and those in other articles you have read. You can then compare the article with others related in topic or methodology when you write your review.

Table 2.2   Preparing to write an article review

Let us now consider one possible way of organizing and structuring the review. This approach divides the review into five sections:

Section 1 gives the full **bibliographic reference** of the article: its author/s, title, journal name, volume, issue, year and page numbers.

Section 2 is the introduction. Here, you should state the topic of the article and the thesis or main idea/purpose of your review. You should also include the audience for whom the article was written, and the assumptions the article appears to make about the reader's background knowledge.

Then, say something about the journal itself. Get a copy from your university library and read the aims and scope of the journal so that you can say whether it is the appropriate journal for this particular article. Finally, mention what type of article this is. Articles can be classified into two types:

- the conceptual article: it supports its thesis mainly by means of logical and **persuasive reasoning**;
- the empirical article: it supports its thesis with substantial evidence normally drawn from research studies.

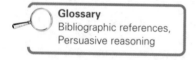

Glossary
Bibliographic references,
Persuasive reasoning

Section 3 is the summary of the article. Remember to provide your reader with only the main points of the content and arguments in it. Your brief summary (no more than 3 paragraphs) should include:

- the problem being addressed;
- if available, the research questions that have prompted the author/s to conduct the experiment or write the argument;
- the solution being proposed and the evidence being provided.

Section 4 is the core of your review. This is the analysis. It is where you show how well you can evaluate the strengths and weaknesses of the article and how clearly you can define your position in relation to the author's. In this section, you should examine whether the article establishes a logical connection between the research questions introduced at the beginning of the article, the evidence presented in the body of the article to answer these questions, and the conclusions it reaches, based on that evidence.

Suppose you were reading an article whose author had wanted to investigate the perceptions a group of women in a given geographical area held about the care received post-natally. You would expect an article like this to be based on data collected from this specific population. You would expect it to describe research methods and data collection instruments appropriate for 'capturing perceptions' (e.g. in-depth interviews). Then, depending on the

Activity 2.3

Read the following introduction of an article review and decide if it is a good example. Here are some questions that may help you decide:

1 Does it include all the necessary bibliographical information?
2 Does it state the topic (of the article) and the purpose (of the review)?
3 Does it mention the audience of the article and the assumptions the writer has made about them?
4 Does it refer to the journal as an appropriate forum for the article?
5 Does it mention what type of article this is?

Aston J, Shi E, Bullôt H, Galway R, Crisp J. (2006). Quantitative evaluation of regular morning meetings aimed at improving work practices associated with effective interdisciplinary communication. *International Journal of Nursing Practice*.

This article reports on a research study which aims to evaluate interdisciplinary surgical morning meetings (SMM) at a ward of a major paediatric hospital. Such meetings were introduced to reduce communication and work process problems among interdisciplinary professionals who provided care for children and their families. The article was written for nurses and doctors working in infants' and toddlers' hospital wards. The writers assume their readers will not only have clinical experience in these wards but will also be aware of the problems of miscommunication and its implications for the children and their families. The journal is an appropriate choice for this empirical article as it publishes contributions that, according to its aims and scope, advance the 'understanding and development of nursing, both as a profession and as an academic discipline'. This review will provide a short description of the study and evaluate its contributions to the existing body of knowledge about interdisciplinary teams in acute-care environments.

Answers See suggested answers on page 191.

data size, you would expect it to generalize results and draw conclusions that might apply to similar contexts. Judging whether it does these things satisfactorily would form the core of your review.

This section should also indicate your **stance** as a reviewer in a critical manner. It should show:

- whether you agree or disagree with the point/points made by the author;
- your reasons for this;

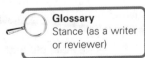

Glossary
Stance (as a writer or reviewer)

- how any weaknesses you have spotted could have been avoided;
- any assumptions that you believe affect the validity of the study.

This section will vary slightly depending on whether you are reviewing a conceptual or an empirical article. If you are working on a conceptual article, this section should include:

- an appreciation of its logic: do the different parts of the article contradict one other? Does the conclusion logically result from the introduction and the arguments in the body?
- a consideration of its coherence: does the line of reasoning follow a coherent development? Does each part naturally lead to the next?
- an analysis of the substance of the article: does the article shed new light on the issues it explores? Does it just summarize previous knowledge or debates?

If you are reviewing an empirical article, you should then look at things such as:

- its clarity: does the article clearly develop its research question/s?
- its literature review: where does the research connect with the existing literature?
- its design: is this the most appropriate way to investigate the research question/s? Are the data collection instruments well-designed? How valid is the study?
- its analysis of the data: are the statistics used appropriate for the type of data? Is the description of qualitative data enough to understand the analysis?
- its discussion and conclusions: are the author's claims clearly justified?
- its ethical considerations and the biases of the authors: have the ethical issues been addressed? Have the authors done anything to minimize their own biases?

Section 5 is the conclusion. Here, you sum up your position in relation to the article and indicate the contributions that the article makes to the field.

There are many different ways in which an article may contribute to advancements in its field; it may:

- look at an old problem from a new perspective;

- provide new results or shed new light on something old;
- suggest new solutions;
- present issues in a way that the relationship between theory and practice is highlighted.

In the conclusion, you should not only state the contributions the article makes, but also why you think its contributions are important or significant.

Activity 2.4

Using the questions in the previous activity and the bulleted points used in various parts of this section, make your own checklist of the things that an effective review article should do. You can divide the checklist into introduction, body and conclusion, for example, which will also help you with the structuring of your reviews.

The argumentative essay: an introduction

This last section of the chapter introduces the argumentative essay. Like the care critique, this is a central genre in nursing and midwifery studies. It's what you'll be doing in the later stages of your course, so we're going to look at it again in Chapter 6. Here, we will consider what argumentation is and analyse the logic and the structure of an argument.

As the cline in Figure 2.2 illustrates, argumentation is different from description. Whereas description entails depicting what something is like or the facts about it (as in the 'room to let' ad), argumentation involves presenting a claim (sometimes called a *thesis*) supported by reasoning and evidence in an attempt to convince readers that the claim or thesis presented is valid (as in the letter to the editor).

An academic argument is also different from a personal opinion in that the latter does not necessarily have to be supported by logical reasoning or evidence. If, for instance, you say 'I don't like the way he treats his patients', you may not need to support your personal opinion with evidence. What is more, if challenged, you could just simply say 'Because I don't.' In academic argumentation, once you have made claim, you need to use evidence to support it.

What is the logic of argumentation? When we plan an argument, we normally think about three things:

- what we assume to be true (e.g. nurses need to learn academic writing to advance their careers);
- our conclusions based on our assumptions (e.g. nurses who can write academic pieces should be better off professionally); and
- the evidence which supports both our assumptions and our conclusions (examples of nurses who have benefited from knowing how to write academically).

The logic of argumentation can be illustrated as in Figure 2.4

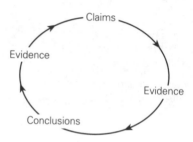

Figure 2.4   The logic of argumentation

It is important to mention here that each of these parts of the logic of an argument is dependent upon the others. Our thesis will obviously affect our conclusions, and if after stating our thesis we find evidence that challenges it, our conclusions will also be challenged. As we saw in connection with the article review, the logic of an argument should follow a coherent development and each part should naturally lead to the next.

As with other pieces of academic writing, when writing an argument you must plan your ideas first. This will help you focus your ideas and make sure they are presented clearly and logically. The guide of Table 2.3 illustrates the typical organization and structuring of an argumentative essay.

As you can see, the overall structure of the argumentative essay follows that of the general academic essay discussed earlier in the chapter. We will discuss this genre in more detail in Chapter 6.

Grammar and English use

In this last section of the chapter you will find some suggestions about how to deal with grammar and language-use problems that many students experience when writing descriptive and critical pieces. If you need more detail

Section	What does it do?
Introduction	States the aim of your essay, presents your claim or thesis, and mentions the reasons given to support your claim.
Statements	As well as including your supporting evidence, the statements discuss evidence that contradicts the argument.
Summary	Presents a brief review of discussion (supporting and contradicting evidence) and balances it, favouring your position.
Conclusion	Re-states the views identified at the beginning of your essay, possibly discusses alternatives, examines implications of the conclusions, and/or makes recommendations based on the conclusions.

Table 2.3   The structure of an argument

Activity 2.5

Read these two short texts; one is more descriptive than the other. Decide which is which, and think of reasons to justify your choice.

Text 1
Many arguments have been advanced in favour of the benefits of returning a patient with a stroke to the open plan unit. These include the positive support reported by the patients and the quality of the follow-up care. However, the advantages of allowing patients with a stroke to stay in the same room have not been fully examined. Many patients with a stroke have reported they would have paid for a private room for critical care. These patients could benefit from having the privacy for themselves and their families that a private room can offer. They could also profit from being closely monitored by the nurse stationed right outside their room.

Text 2
Equipping a room to the standards required for providing critical care involves making many decisions. After recovery, the patient will have to be allowed to stay in the same room. This will reduce patient transport and lower exposure to infections. Nurses' stations will have to be positioned outside the room for easy access and monitoring, while favouring patient privacy at the same time.

Answers See suggested answers on page 191.

on any of these topics, see the Glossary of Key Terms and the list of Further Readings and Resources at the end of the book.

The language of description

In Table 2.4 you will find words (verbs, adjectives, and adverbs) that are frequently used in descriptions. You can use these words to talk about facts and describe what things or persons are like. The table also shows the functions of these words (what you can use them for), their connection with academic writing (the types of writing where you can use them) and some examples.

Word class	Functions	Types of writing	Example
Relating verbs (e.g. be, have, there is, there are)	Definitions, describing features, providing details, making comparisons.	Descriptive record keeping, background information in a case or care critique, providing evidence, describing facts in an argument.	The patient **was** administered 4,000 U standard heparin intravenously before placement of an arterial cross-clamp at 9:32 am.
Action verbs (e.g. discover, report, show, state, compare, contrast)	Describing events, reporting, instructions, making comparisons, describing findings, describing graphs.	Background information in a case or care critique, describing research findings, describing facts in an argument.	The study **reported** an increase in the number of patients who self-refer to hospitals.
Describing words (e.g. essential, informed, static)	Making a description of a person or thing more precise.	More precise description of a person or event.	Midwives play an **essential** role in helping the **pregnant** smoker to make **informed** decisions.
Words that describe actions (e.g. well, slowly, hard)	Making a description of an action more precise.	More precise description of how something was done.	The information leaflets were given out to all patients **effectively**.

Table 2.4   Verbs, adjectives and adverbs used in description

The language of argumentation

In this second table, Table 2.5, you will find words (verbs, adverbs and connectives) that are frequently used in writing critical genres such as the article review, the care critique and argumentative essays. The table shows the functions of these words, and some examples.

Word class	Functions	Example
Acknowledging verbs (e.g. admit, recognize)	To admit limitations or incompleteness.	We have to **admit** two main limitations in this study.
Comparing verbs (e.g. correspond to, compare with)	To draw a comparison between ideas or arguments.	His position **compares** favourably with that of his predecessors.
Emphasizing verbs (e.g. insist, reiterate, remark, stress)	To provide emphasis to a point/idea in an argument, or the argument itself.	She **insists** that these are fundamental considerations relating to clinical care.
Establishing verbs (e.g. demonstrate, prove, solve, fail)	To establish that someone or something has or hasn't been successful at demonstrating something.	This has **demonstrated** that not all patients favour moving to an open plan unit after they have recovered.
Positioning verbs (e.g. claim, hold the view, recommend, suggest)	To show the writer's position, discuss it and/or challenge it.	This seems to **suggest** that the writer considers that most of these events could have been prevented.
Emphasizing adverbs (e.g. convincingly, conclusively, definitely, forcefully, successfully)	To emphasise how something was done.	They have **forcefully** made the case that units should be fully equipped to provide the best possible care.

Table 2.5 Verbs, adverbs and connectives used in argumentation

Revising the objectives of this chapter

Tick those objectives you feel you have achieved and review those you have not yet managed to accomplish. Then, complete the **Achievement Chart** at the back of the book.

In this chapter, you have learnt to:

- [ ] recognise the difference between description and argumentation

- [ ] identify the main academic genres in nursing and midwifery

- [ ] understand the purpose and the structure of these genres

- [ ] identify main language items used in descriptive and critical writing

3 Writing Processes in Academic Writing

At the end of this chapter, you should be able to:

- ▶ recognize the nature and stages of the reflective process
- ▶ identify different critical thinking processes
- ▶ understand the principles of critical evaluation of evidence
- ▶ identify key language items used in reflective and critical writing

● Reflection and the reflective process

Chapters 1 and 2 have laid down the foundations of academic writing. Chapter 1 explored three basic issues in academic writing: planning, organizing and para-graphing and Chapter 2 built on those principles to deal with more specific genres such as the care critique, the journal article and the argumentative essay. This chapter deals with reflection and critical thinking, two specific processes you will need to write other genres such as the reflective essay in Chapter 4. The chapter starts exploring the nature and stages of the reflective process and then moves on to analyse the principles of critical thinking.

In this section of the chapter, you will analyse reflection as a concept and as a process.

Let us start by looking at some phrases connected with reflection as a concept. Complete the spidergram below with three words or phrases you usually associate with 'reflection'. One has been given as an example.

Glossary
Reflection

You probably included ideas such as 'learning from past experience', 'evaluating what happened', 'applying practical wisdom', 'examining what was done', 'getting better prepared for the future' and 'empowering'. All these ideas have to do with reflection.

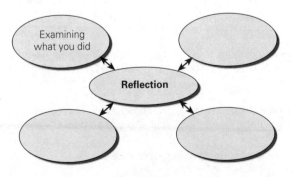

Simply defined, reflection means learning from what you do so you can be better prepared for the future. Through reflection you can learn to change aspects of yourself, your professional practice, or both. Reflection can be seen as a bridge that connects past and present experiences to decide what future actions you need to take (Durgahee, 1996).

Donald Schon (1987) distinguished between 'reflection-on-action' and 'reflection-in-action'. Reflection-**on**-action is about looking back at an experience or event. Reflection-**in**-action is associated with thinking about something while you're still doing it.

In this chapter you will be concerned with **reflection-on-action** – that is, with examining a past event so you can learn how to do better in the future.

Reflection-on-action

This learning experience has three aspects to it, matched by three action stages as illustrated in Table 3.1.

Figure 3.1 shows the reflection-on-action process. Notice that the reflective process is cyclical rather than linear. Today you revisit yesterday's events, but tomorrow you will need to revise today's experiences. This is the essence of reflection as a process for professional development and as the basis for becoming a reflective professional.

Reflection-on-action examines past events or experiences from a critical perspective. Remember that it is a learning experience that aims to improve the weaknesses in the professional practice of the person who reflects.

This means that reflection is a *critical* and *evaluative* process. It is not a *descriptive* process. This critical and evaluative process is clearly manifested in the reflective essay, which we will discuss in more depth in Chapter 4.

Aspect	Action
Reflexivity: looking at how 'self' has developed throughout time.	You revisit or describe a past event or experience and think about the people involved in it.
Understanding: gaining insights as to how and why things happened.	You examine what happened, why it happened, and how it could be done differently.
Empowerment: being able to change things in the future.	You then decide on a course of action that will help you do things better next time.

Table 3.1 Aspects of the learning experience

Let us now examine the different stages of reflection-on-action as outlined above. Researchers have put forward many conceptual models of reflection-on-action, the three best-known models being those developed by Van Manen (1977), Gibbs (1988) and Durgahee (1996). Van Manen's is a general model that details reflection as a process for professional advancement. It includes three different levels of reflection: the evaluation of a given performance, the analysis of its consequences and the critical examination of its associated issues.

Both Gibbs' and Durgahee's models work at a more practicable level. Gibbs' model is probably the most widely cited in nursing and midwifery. It comprises the following stages:

- description: what happened, what your feelings were at the time;
- evaluation: what was good and bad about the situation;
- analysis: what sense you can make of it;
- conclusion: what else could have been done;
- action: what you would do next time around.

Durgahee divides reflection into three levels:

- macro level: the actual recall of the experience;
- meso level: the identification of its associated issues;
- micro level: the understanding of the experience based on feelings and personal views.

As with most conceptualizations, these models have their limitations; however, they represent three strong theoretical frameworks for developing the critical skills needed for reflection.

For each of the three stages in the reflection-on-action process illustrated in Figure 3.1, there are some **critical skills** you will need to develop. These

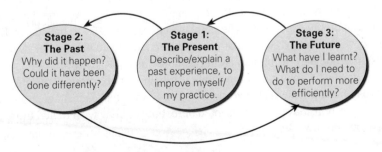

Figure 3.1 The reflection-on-action cycle

critical skills are highlighted in italics in the following description of the reflective process:

- The **first stage** involves not only explaining the experience and issues identified in it but also *exploring preconceptions* and *assumptions* about it.
- The **second stage** analyses what happened and the reasons why it happened but also deals with *questioning/challenging the preconceptions* revisited in the first stage.
- The **third stage** is the actual reflection, by which you not only examine what has been learnt and what needs yet to be learnt but *identify learning needs* and *plan concrete actions* to resolve future conflicts.

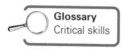

Glossary
Critical skills

Let us analyse the critical skills involved in each step in more depth. After explaining the main issues which resulted from the experience you revisited in the first stage, you need to explore the preconceptions and assumptions made at the time of the experience. It is important to notice here that exploring preconceptions and assumption does not mean finding a justification for them, but rather producing an objective analysis of what lies behind them.

The second stage involves challenging these preconceived ideas. Are they still valid? Do they need to be modified? If they do, how can they be modified? What would be the most appropriate way of modifying the preconceived ideas identified? This stage is more analytic in nature than the first one.

The third stage is the most critical. In this last stage you should adopt an objective perspective on the experience and on your feelings about it, making a connection between what you have learnt from this and the actions that you plan to take for the future.

Table 3.2 on pages 50 and 51 is a summary of the issues involved in each of the three stages and the skills the student in the case above would need to reflect upon the experience. The numbers in brackets refer to the stages; the reflective skills required are in italics and given in square brackets. How does this table compare with the answers you provided in Activity 3.1?

As Table 3.2 shows, key questions can help you go through the different stages to identify the reflective skills you need to use in each stage. Some of these questions have been presented here, but you may wish to add more or develop your own set.

Activity 3.1

Read the following short case and think of how the student involved in it could reflect upon the experience. Then complete the chart with your ideas on the issues she should identify at each stage and the reflective skills needed for each of the stages.

On her first clinical placement, a student nurse was asked by her placement supervisor to care for a client in a wheelchair. She hadn't done this before and she wasn't sure she could manage. Nevertheless, she decided not to tell her supervisor that she had no experience with anyone in a wheelchair. She was asked to take the client to radiology for an x-ray. Before pushing the chair, the student wanted to make sure that the client had her feet on the foot rest. She pushed the foot rest into position and, without realizing, she hurt the client's leg.

Stage	Issues to identify	Critical skills needed
1 **Explaining &** **Exploring**	Explaining the experience:	Exploring preconceptions/ assumptions:
2 **Analysing &** **Challenging**	Analysing what happened and why; how it could have been different:	Challenging preconceptions/ assumptions:
3 **Examining,** **Identifying &** **Planning**	Examining what has been learnt:	Identifying learning needs/ planning actions:

Answers See suggested answers in Table 3.2.

● The principles of critical thinking

Being able to reflect on your practice is an important part of the broader process of becoming a critical thinker. In this part of the chapter we will look at the principles of critical thinking and see how you can develop your own critical thinking abilities. Being a good critical thinker means you can assess the arguments presented by other people to see if they are logical, well

Stages	Issues	Skills
Stage 1: Explaining & Exploring	**What happened? (1)** 1 It was the first time the student had to provide care for a person in a wheelchair. 2 The student did not say how she was feeling about the request. 3 The wheelchair footrest hurt the client's leg. **Context (1)** 4 The student's first clinical placement. 5 The hospital ward, the radiology department. **Who was involved? (1)** 6 The placement supervisor. 7 The student nurse. 8 The client.	**What assumptions did they make? (1)** [exploring assumptions] 9 Supervisor: The student knew what to do and how to do it. 10 The student: She could eventually handle the task.
Stage 2: Analysing & Challenging	**Why did it happen? (2)** 11 The student didn't tell the supervisor she had never provided care for a person in a wheelchair. 12 The supervisor failed to check.	**Did the assumptions prove right? (2** [challenging assumptions] 14 For the supervisor. 15 For the student nurse.

thought out, and properly supported with relevant evidence. It is an ability that you can use when you read as well as when you listen to someone presenting a point of view or proposing a course of action.

Stella Cottrell (2005: 2) defines critical thinking as 'a complex process of deliberation which includes a wide range of skills and attitudes'. This implies that you can identify these skills and evaluate how good you are at each of them so you can improve any weak areas.

When you are assessing someone else's arguments, good critical thinking includes being able to:

Stages	Issues	Skills
	Could it have been done differently? (2) 13 Yes, the supervisor could have taught the student how to handle the situation.	**Do the assumptions need to be changed? (2)** 16 Do the supervisor's assumptions need to be changed? If so, how can they be changed? 17 Do the student's assumptions need to be changed? If so, how?
Stage 3: Examining, Identifying & Planning	**What should the student have learnt from this experience? (3)** 18 Effective communication is extremely important in caring for patients. 19 Decisions should be informed and based on knowledge and experience.	**What does the student still need to learn? (3)** [*identifying learning need*] 20 To express her feelings, especially when she is doing something for the first time. 21 To get support when she is doing things she feels she is not fully trained for. 22 To gauge the possible consequences of her actions. 23 To learn to make more informed decisions. **Future action (3)** [*Planning concrete actions*] 24 To learn ways of expressing feelings. 25 To get trained in handling and moving patients.

Table 3.2   The reflective stages

- identify other people's positions, arguments and conclusions;
- evaluate the evidence for alternative points of view;
- weigh up opposing arguments and evidence fairly;
- draw conclusions about whether arguments are valid and justifiable, based on good evidence and sensible assumptions.

When you are writing an essay or presenting your point of view, critical thinking allows you to present an argument in a structured, clear, well-reasoned way that convinces others.

These skills and attitudes can be seen to fall into three different phases which are essential to the critical thinking process: **identifying, evaluating** and **presenting**.

These phases may seem linear, but in actual practice they may occur more than once in a cyclical manner. For instance, you may need to revisit the position that other people have put forward as you realize that some of the assumptions on which their argument was based are false.

What does each of these phases involve?

Phase 1: Identifying positions, arguments and conclusions

To recognize people's positions, you will need to identify:

- how they position themselves in their argument;
- what positions by others they endorse or do not endorse;
- what possible biases their arguments present.

The way people use language can provide you with valuable help to recognize their positions. Some questions you can use to discover a writer's or speaker's position, for example, include:

- Are they positioning themselves as part of the issues analysed? As an insider? Or an objective outsider? What grammatical person (e.g. he, she, they) do they use? What grammatical structures (e.g. impersonal 'it') do they employ?
- What does the writer or speaker agree with? What do they disagree with? What verbs do they use to mark endorsement or lack of it (e.g. these authors have advanced influential..., these writers have ignored...)?
- Are the person's own biases recognized? Do they use language that indicates this (e.g. I intend to follow...)?

Identifying people's arguments at this stage is also connected with how they structure the information in the arguments. You need to identify the claim that serves as a starting point for their argument, how their claim is supported and what conclusion or conclusions they draw as a result (see also Chapter 6).

Consider, for example, the following claim in an article on encouraging pregnant women to stop smoking:

> Smoking cessation during pregnancy is unsuccessful because support to the pregnant woman is only occasional and lacks structure.

If you identify this as the writer's main argument, you should expect a critique of current systems of support, based on evidence. You should also find some conclusions and recommendations about how smoking cessation during pregnancy can be made more effective. Coupled with this structural recognition, you should also identify some strategies that can make the writer's argument more persuasive. Some of these strategies involve:

- presenting the opposing argument first;
- using **transition markers** that indicate an opposing view (e.g. 'however', 'nevertheless'), which can also help highlight the writer's own argument;
- contrasting the weaknesses of the first argument (usually the opposing argument) with the strengths of the writer's argument.

Phase 2: Evaluating evidence and arguments

This is a central stage in the critical thinking process. Here, you need to consider whether the writer or speaker has presented a balanced picture by offering evidence to both support and counter his/her views. Other important aspects to consider are the value of the evidence used, whether the logic of the argument is flawed, and whether the conclusion is logical. Some questions you can use to evaluate evidence and arguments include:

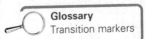

Glossary
Transition markers

- Does the writer present a balanced picture of the issue/s by including opposing views and arguments? How balanced is the presentation?
- How strong is the evidence presented to support the claims being made? Is it closely related to the argument? Or is it only indirectly linked? Is it practice-based? Is it research-based?
- Is there a logical relationship between the different parts (claim, evidence, and conclusion) of the argument?
- Does the conclusion develop logically from the issues explored and the evidence presented?

Phase 3: The presentation of the argument

This phase is crucial for evaluating other people's arguments. Like identifying, presenting combines structural as well as logical elements. The logical elements are connected with how well reasoned and well balanced the argument is. The structural elements have to do with the clarity and structure. Questions to examine the presentation of an argument may include:

- Does the presentation contribute to persuading the reader that the argument is valid?
- Are the arguments presented in a well-thought-out and clearly planned manner?
- Does the presentation follow a logical order?
- Does the writer use language effectively to support his/her logical order (e.g. using connectives such as 'first', 'finally', 'on the other hand')?

Activity 3.2

Applying the three phases of critical thinking (identifying, evaluating and presenting), analyse the following short text. Can you recognize any of the critical strategies discussed so far? Use some of the questions suggested for each phase to help you.

Many studies have produced inconclusive evidence in relation to the efficacy of the support that smokers receive during pregnancy (e.g. Kelley *et al.* 2001; Kelly *et al.*, 2001; Melvin *et al.* 2000; Melvin & Gaffney, 2004). Several of these studies suggest that brief interventions do not significantly contribute to smoking cessation during pregnancy (Fiore *et al.*, 2000; Lumley *et al.*, 2004). Lawrence *et al.*; (2005: p. 115), for example, have forcefully concluded that 'in-pregnancy programmes may have immediate benefits to the foetus, but do not influence the smoking outcomes of mothers in the medium term.' This seems to indicate that smoking cessation in pregnancy is unsuccessful because support to the pregnant woman is only occasional and lacks structure. Programmes of sustained support would need to be implemented so as to help smokers not only during pregnancy but also after giving birth. These programmes should then be structured in such a way as to offer both in-pregnancy and postpartum support. Combined strategies have been suggested as a successful element of these programmes. Some of the in-pregnancy strategies may include providing information leaflets on the risks of maternal smoking to the foetus and the infant, helping to set a quit date, and teaching cognitive and behavioural strategies for stopping. After-pregnancy strategies should include control of the levels of nicotine, provision of rewards and peer support groups.

Answers See suggested answers on page 192.

● Critical analysis of evidence

In the previous section you examined how to identify a writer's or speaker's claims and purpose, and how to evaluate the consistency and worth of his/her arguments. Another important skill in critical thinking is being able to evaluate the sources of evidence someone has used to support their argument. Although this critical analysis is important for all kinds of sources of evidence, it becomes of paramount importance when you have to examine electronic sources (see Chapter 1).

In this section, you will examine two different, though interrelated, ways of evaluating sources. You will first look at the *quality* of the sources and then at their *relevance*.

Determining the quality of the sources used to support an argument is fundamental as their quality will determine the quality of the argument itself. Sources in an argument are like the foundations in a house. If the foundations are not properly laid, the rest of the structure may collapse.

Typical questions you may ask when analysing the *quality* of the sources used to support an argument include:

- Who wrote the material? What professional affiliation do they have? Have they written on the subject before? Are they cited by others?
- When was the evidence published?
- In the case of evidence found in books, is the book a new edition? Has the new edition been (substantially) revised?
- Who published the material?
- What kind of publication is it? Is it an internationally-known journal? Is it a local newspaper?
- Who was the material written for? Who was its intended audience? Was it written for the general public?
- Was the content presented in a well-reasoned manner? Are there flaws?
- How much does the content cover (breadth and depth of coverage)?
- What contribution does the content make to the issue/s being discussed?

The *relevance* of source material is related to the importance of the information to develop the writer's claims. The questions you need to ask to examine the relevance of the sources include:

- Are the claims and supporting evidence closely related? Are the claims too general?
- Does some of the evidence challenge the claims?
- Is the evidence strong enough for the writer to have a case?
- Does the conclusion develop logically from the claims and the supporting evidence?

Activity 3.3

Look at the following sources of evidence. Can you evaluate them in terms of their quality? You will need to do a library or internet search to find more information about them before you can decide on their quality. Use the suggested questions of this section if you need guidance.

1 Maslin-Prothero, S. (ed.) (1997) *Baillière's Study Skills for Nurses*. London: Baillière Tindall in association with the Royal College of Nursing.

2 Terry Lawrence, P. Aveyard, K. K. Cheng, C. Griffin, C. Johnson and E. Croghan (2005). 'Does stage-based smoking cessation advice in pregnancy result in long-term quitters? 18-month postpartum follow-up of a randomized controlled trial', *Addiction*, vol. 100/1: 107–16.

3 'Evaluating Sources of Information', *Online Writing Lab*, Purdue University. Available at http://owl.english.purdue.edu/workshops/hypertext/EvalSrcW/, accessed on 8 March 2006.

4 Spiegel, R. (2004). *Psychopharmacology: An Introduction*. 4th edn. Chichester, West Sussex: John Wiley & Sons, Ltd.

Answers See suggested answers on page 192.

Reflection and critical thinking are cognitive processes that require specific language and grammar when you need to talk or write about them. The process of reflection, for instance, requires that you keep the right sequence of tenses when you refer to the past event upon which you are reflecting, your present reflection and the future actions you intend to take. Similarly, critical thinking tends to be associated with certain verbs such as 'analyse' and 'synthesize' and certain structures which you can use to show your stance as a writer. These issues are explored in the next section.

Grammar and English use

In this section you will find suggestions about how to deal with some grammar and language-use problems that many students have when using reflection and critical skills. If you need more detail on any of these topics, see the Glossary of Key Terms and the list of Further Readings and Resources at the end of the book.

Verbs connected to 'reflection'

Table 3.3 on the following page shows some verbs that recur when discussing reflection. It also shows associated words that you can use to, for instance, avoid repetition or create cohesion in your texts (see Chapter 1). Some examples of how you can use them are also given.

Tense sequence for reflection

When writing a reflective essay, keeping the right sequence of tenses (present, past, future) may prove problematic. Below are some key things you should remember about tense sequence.

Present descriptions: present time in real situations (not hypothetical or imaginary ones) can be described by:

- simple present (The morning shift for nurses **starts** at 6.00 am).
- present progressive (The patient **is being** diagnosed).

Present tenses are normally used to describe the event or situation upon which we want to reflect. How these tenses combine depends on the logical sequence of events. For example, the present perfect (e.g. have gone, has decided) has a connection with the past (an action that started some time in the past) and usually means the action is not finished. It may be necessary as background information to a present event:

> He *has been taken* to the operating room where he *is being operated* on for tendon rupture.

Present descriptions tend to connect with the future by means of the future simple tense (will):

> After the nurses finish with the admission routine, the patient *will* be sent to the A&E unit.

Past recounts: past events can also be described by a number of past tenses:

- simple past (The treatment **was** a success.)
- past progressive (They **were organizing** the patient's records when they were called to a staff meeting.)

Verb	Common accompanying words	Example
Assess	<u>Noun</u>: assessment <u>Adverbs</u>: accurately, correctly, fully, properly <u>Similar words</u>: appraise, evaluate, estimate	Reflecting upon the experience provided her with an opportunity to accurately **assess** the situation in the ward.
Assume	<u>Noun</u>: assumption <u>Adverbs</u>: naturally, reasonably, safely <u>Similar words</u>: presume, suppose	She first **assumed** that nurses were familiar with the side effects of all drugs.
Attend to	<u>Noun</u>: attention <u>Adverbs</u>: constantly, carefully <u>Similar words</u>: deal with, take care of	In the first place, it was necessary to **attend to** every one of her needs constantly.
Challenge	<u>Noun</u>: challenge <u>Adverbs</u>: effectively, forcefully, seriously, (un)successfully <u>Similar words</u>: contest, question	Her initial assumptions were seriously **challenged** by the facts she later collected.
Evaluate	<u>Noun</u>: evaluation <u>Adverbs</u>: carefully, constantly, critically, fully, properly, systematically, thoroughly <u>Similar words</u>: assess, estimate	His assumptions were systematically **evaluated** against the sources associated with smoking cessation during pregnancy.
Explore	<u>Noun</u>: exploration <u>Adverbs</u>: carefully, briefly, extensively, fully, systematically, thoroughly	In the second stage, they had to **explore** all the possible alternatives before they could make a final decision.

- past perfect (They **had finished** completing the admission form when the patient collapsed.)

In some cases two past actions can be described by using the simple past without creating confusion in the reader. For example:

> The nurse *managed* to finish the admission form before the patient *collapsed*.

Verb	Common accompanying words	Example
Identify	<u>Noun</u>: identification <u>Adverbs</u>: accurately, clearly, (in)correctly, positively <u>Similar words</u>: distinguish, single (out)	It is essential to **identify** the assumptions lying behind one's own actions.
Involve	<u>Noun</u>: involvement <u>Adverbs</u>: actively, directly, inevitably, typically <u>Similar words</u>: entail, include	The problem **involves** all people connected with his care: his nurse, his social worker and his family.
Perform	<u>Noun</u>: performance <u>Adverbs</u>: adequately, effectively, efficiently, <u>Similar words</u>: accomplish, achieve	You can learn a great deal from examining in retrospect how your peers **performed**.
Plan	<u>Noun</u>: plan <u>Adverbs</u>: carefully, intelligibly, meticulously, systematically <u>Similar words</u>: chart, project, map (out)	Based on your own past learning experiences, you can carefully **plan** further actions to be better prepared for the future.
Reflect (up)on	<u>Noun</u>: reflection <u>Adverbs</u>: fully, thoroughly <u>Similar words</u>: think	This essay will **reflect** upon the most central issues associated with primary care.

Table 3.3 Verbs used in reflective texts

This is usually the case when you use words such as 'before' and 'after' to join the two actions. But notice the difference in meaning between these two versions of the same example:

1 The nurse *had finished* the admission form when the patient *collapsed*.
2 The nurse *finished* the admission form when the patient *collapsed*.

The past perfect (*had finished*) in (1) is used to indicate that this is the first of the two actions. The simple past (*finished*) in (2) is used to indicate that both activities happened at almost the same time.

To indicate future in the past we use 'would' instead of will:

> The doctor thought the patient's heart would not restart.

Future actions: actions in the future can be expressed by:

- the simple future (They **will** finish their midwifery programme in 6 months.)
- the present progressive to indicate an arrangement (I **am seeing** my placement supervisor next week.)
- 'going to' to indicate a future plan (The student **is going to** get some training in handling and moving patients.)

Verbs connected to 'critical thinking'

Table 3.4 on the following page shows some verbs used in connection with critical thinking, words that are commonly associated with these verbs (collocations) and some examples.

● Showing your stance

A writer's stance can be defined as his/her position in relation to the subject matter of his/her writing and how he/she relates with the audience. For example, in a sentence like 'helping women make informed decisions is a fundamental aspect of the role of the midwife', you can see that the writer views the subject matter (helping women make informed decisions) as an essential part of the role of the midwife. In a sentence like 'Most readers will certainly appreciate the importance of effective communication in providing nursing care for patients', you can see that by addressing the audience directly (most readers will) the writer is establishing a relationship with them. Also if you carefully look at the writer's choice of words (most, certainly, appreciate, importance, effective), you can see how the writer relates with the subject matter. Similarly, you can interpret other people's stance as writers by the verb you use to report their words. If, for example, you write 'Brown (2004) says that ...' you are just reporting but not interpreting Brown's words as when you write 'Brown (2004) denies/criticizes/ suggests that ...'

Thus, 'showing your stance' as a writer means showing how certain you are about what you're claiming, how you feel about it, or how strongly you

Verb	Connected words	Example
Analyse	answers, arguments, evidence, ideas, methods, preferences, relationships, theories, etc.	This essay will **analyse** the relationship between these two aspects.
Be	accurate, active, analytical, consistent, evaluative, logical, open-minded, precise, rational, systematic, etc.	Their argument **is** a systematic attempt to end world poverty and ill-health.
Differentiate	attitudes, facts, fallacies, ideas, opinions, truth, etc.	It is important to be able to **differentiate** facts from opinions.
Draw	attention, conclusions, distinctions, inferences, lessons, plans, etc.	Its ultimate aim is to try and **draw** lessons from these changes.
Evaluate	accuracy, arguments, assumptions, authenticity, beliefs, evidence, viewpoints, worth, etc.	He has always been good at **evaluating** the authenticity of other people's claims.
Identify	arguments, ideas, differences, positions, similarities , etc.	The next section of this critique will **identify** the differences and similarities between the two methods.
Interpret	meanings, experiences, information, results, significance, sources, etc.	They failed to **interpret** the results of the study in the light of the research questions posed at the beginning of their article.
Weigh up	advantages, (opposing) arguments, disadvantages, risks, etc.	Risks should always be **weighed** up against the benefits that clients may get.

Table 3.4   Verbs used in critical thinking texts

support someone else's opinion. Here are some examples of how you can show your stance:

1   The results of the study **are** inconclusive.
2   The results of the study **seem** inconclusive.

3 The results of the study **may seem** inconclusive.
4 The results of the study **might look** inconclusive.

Sentences (1)-(4) show different degrees of certainty, from most certain to least certain. That is, they show how positive you are about the claim you're making. By using words or phrases such as 'seem', 'may', 'probably', 'appear to be', 'might', you can indicate a more tentative stance than when you use the verb 'to be' for instance, as in (1) above.

5 The **deadly** virus has reached continental Europe.

Adjectives (e.g. deadly) and adverbs (e.g. forcefully) give the reader an indication of where you stand in relation to the facts described. In sentence (5) above, the writer is showing his/her position in respect of the spread of the virus.

Your choice of verbs also shows your position as a writer with regard to other people's ideas or arguments. Notice the difference in 'strength' of support to what others have expressed given by 'suggest' in (6) and 'confirm' in (7).

6 Brown (2003) **suggests** that the contradictory results in these two studies have been produced by the different research methods used.
7 Ellis (1994) **has confirmed** that women who suffer from postpartum depression find support groups extremely useful.

Another way of showing your stance is by referring to previous work that has influenced yours, establishing similarities and differences between them as shown in example (8) below.

8 This essay follows Gibbs' pioneering examination of reflection as the basis for professional development. Unlike Gibbs', the present framework, however, aims at...

Revising the objectives of this chapter

Tick those objectives you feel you have achieved and review those you have not yet managed to accomplish. Then complete the **Achievement Chart** at the back of the book.

In this chapter, you have learnt to:

- ☐ recognize the nature and stages of the reflective process

- ☐ identify different critical thinking processes

- ☐ understand the principles of critical evaluation of evidence

- ☐ identify key language items used in reflection and critical writing

Part Two

Writing Genres in Nursing and Midwifery

This second part consists of four 'how to' chapters that will help you apply the principles of academic writing you examined in Part One. In this part, you will study how to write a reflective essay, a care critique, an argument, and four other common nursing and midwifery genres: the action plan, the care plan, the portfolio, the report, and the research proposal.

Chapter 4: How to write a reflective essay

The reflective essay is often one of the first pieces of writing that nursing and midwifery students are required to write. This chapter will show you how to apply the theoretical principles outlined in the previous chapter to develop the different sections of the reflective essay.

Chapter 5: How to write a care critique

Chapter 5 focuses on the process and the product of critiquing. It starts by examining what is involved in writing a care critique, and how it is organized and structured. It then shows how the final product should reflect the critique of the care in its conclusion and recommendations.

Chapter 6: How to write an argument

This chapter opens with exercises to help you differentiate between opinion and argument. It then presents practical ways of identifying the strength of an argument, followed by considerations about structuring arguments effectively. Finally, the chapter identifies main language items that are commonly used in argumentative writing.

• Chapter 7: How to write other genres

Chapter 7 introduces other common genres that you may have to master. The chapter first examines action plans, care plans and portfolios; it then focuses on academic and professional reports. The chapter moves on to analyse the research proposal that you will have to present for your dissertation, and finally it explores how to plan and get organized to write an undergraduate dissertation.

4 How to Write a Reflective Essay

At the end of this chapter, you should be able to:

▶ plan a reflective essay appropriately
▶ identify an effective way of introducing reflective essays
▶ recognize the structure of body paragraphs to support introductions
▶ recognize ways of producing an effective conclusion
▶ identify the style of the reflective essay

● Planning the reflective essay

In Chapter 3 we analysed the nature and the structure of the reflective process. In this chapter we will examine how this process can be used to plan a reflective essay. The reflective essay is an analytic piece of writing. This means that when you write a reflective essay, you need most of the reflective and critical skills examined in Chapter 3. It also means that description will be used as background information but it will not be the focus of a reflective essay.

Let us start by drawing a comparison between description and reflection based on two experiences on clinical placement. Read the main differences between these two processes as illustrated in Table 4.1.

When planning a reflective essay, you will find it useful to devise a table like Table 4.1, where you can list the main differences between description and reflection in relation to the experience you want to analyse. As this table shows, description is concerned with the factual – the reality around the experience. Reflection, on the other hand, has to do with evaluating the event so that it becomes a learning experience.

Your reflective essay will have to combine the description of the facts that made up the event or experience with your 'reflective evaluation' of it. Remember, however, that description will be a small part of the reflective essay. It will only be used to set the scene or provide the background information upon which your evaluation will rest. You will have to describe the event, but you will also need to demonstrate how and what you have learnt from it.

Here are some further steps you will want to consider when planning the structure of your reflective essays:

● examine the essay question;
● read the marking criteria if available;

Past experience	Description	Reflection
A student nurse on a recent clinical placement	The physical environment where he was (the ward, the beds, the clients), who he talked to (supervisors, clients, nurses, other students), what he did (what he was told or asked to do).	How he felt at the time, what he learnt from the experience, what he discovered he didn't know, what perceptions he had before the placement (were they confirmed/ challenged?), what he plans to do about his lacks, what skills he has developed/ needs to acquire.
A student helping a midwife with a breastfeeding educational campaign	The physical environment where she was (the room, the clients), who she interviewed, what the midwife did with the women, what was said, the procedures followed.	How she felt about the experience and the procedures, what she learnt, her assumptions at the time, what she needs for her development as a future midwife.

Table 4.1   Description vs. reflection

- identify the event or experience upon which you will reflect;
- make sure you maintain the anonymity and confidentiality of the patients, clients, staff and institutions involved;
- jot down notes that briefly describe the experience (you can draw up a table here or draw a mind-map or a concept map);
- make a note of the main issues you have been able to identify in relation to the experience;
- think of ways in which you can relate these main issues to the literature (sources);
- jot down some further notes that reflect your understanding of the issues identified, and the insights you gained from the experience;
- think of ways in which you can relate insights you have gained to the literature (sources);
- make notes as to how you will make the connection between theory and practice clear; and
- note down how you plan to discuss your future personal and professional development needs.

Activity 4.1

Read the following account of a past experience a student midwife went through. Use the chart below to differentiate between description and reflection in the account.

A mother's perception of milk insufficiency seems to be one of the most common reasons for discontinuing breastfeeding. As a student, I assisted a midwife in providing care for Isobel, a prima-gravida, two days after normal delivery of her baby. We visited Isobel in her home, a terraced house in the Borough of Haringey, London. Isobel had become very anxious about breastfeeding as she reported her baby did not seem to be getting enough milk and demanded to be breastfed all the time. Isobel felt she needed to start complementing breast milk. Having made sure the baby was latching properly, I told the client that it was normal for some babies to require to be fed all the time. As a way of building the mother's confidence and to avoid discontinuing breastfeeding, the midwife explained to her the supply and demand nature of breast milk. Isobel needed to have as much information as possible to make informed decisions. This would also help to lower her anxiety level. This made the writer realize the importance for new mothers to get consistent supervision and breastfeeding advice.

Experience	Description	Reflection

Answers See suggested answers on page 193.

These structural points will show your reader that after the experience you:

- have developed into a more reflective person (reflexivity);
- have gained new insights (understanding); and
- are now able to change things for the future (empowerment).

● Examining introductions

In Chapter 1 we examined the basic elements in essay introductions, and this section of the chapter will analyse other possible elements in the organization and structure of introductions in reflective essays. Remember that introductions are a fundamental part of any essay as they represent the map of the territory the reader will explore.

When readers of your reflective essay finish reading your introduction, they should also be able to answer the four basic questions for any type of essay:

- What is the essay about?
- What exactly does the essay focus on?
- Why is it important to analyse this?
- How will the issues identified be developed?

You may sometimes need to include other pieces of information in the introduction, especially when you are writing a longer essay. Apart from the information provided by the answers to these four questions, your introduction may also need to include:

- A **transition** between the topic and the focus. When the topic is too broad and the focus too narrow, you will need to add one or two transition sentences to make the text flow more smoothly.
- **Definitions** of terms. When you use terms that are controversial or upon which consensus has not yet been reached, you will need to define exactly how you will use them.
- **Reference** to models. In the case of the reflective essay, you may need to state the model of reflection (e.g. Gibbs, 1988) you will follow.

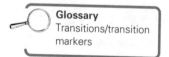
Glossary
Transitions/transition markers

Let us consider two examples of introductions that include these other pieces of information. The first example includes a definition (**D**), a transition (**T**) and a reference to a model (**M**). The second example includes a longer transition (**T**). The first develops the question,

What have you learnt from your recent clinical placement?

and the second answers,

How has your experience in helping the professional activity of a midwife helped you develop new insights?

Example 1 introduction

Reflection has been identified as an extremely useful skill for nurses (Durgahee, 1996; Johns, 1996; Mountford & Rogers, 1996). Schon (1991), for example, defines reflection as learning from events during a practical professional experience (**D**). Clinical placements also offer a unique opportunity for learning through reflection (**T**). Following Gibbs' (1988) cycle of reflection (**M**), this essay will discuss two areas that the writer has been able to identify as needing development for his future professional activity. The first of these is knowledge of the multidimensional nature of pain. The second relates to pain assessment tools, especially in relation to postoperative pain.

Example 2 introduction

Reflection is considered an appropriate vehicle for the analysis of professional practice. This analysis helps professionals understand the nature of their work and adopt a critical approach to their professional activity (Gould & Masters, 2004). Student midwives can also learn from reflecting upon the professional practice of others when, for example, they shadow a midwife on her daily practice on the ward (**T**). This essay reflects on the insights gained in helping the professional activity of a midwife. It first explores the nature and process of reflection. It then examines how reflection has provided the basis for developing new insights into professional midwifery practice. The essay finally recommends future actions to enhance the development of the professional skills of the student midwife.

● Reflection and the body of the essay

The reflection process will find its home in the body of your reflective essay. This means that the body of the reflective essay will contain the different stages of the reflective process we examined in Chapter 3. It will present:

- a description of what happened and what your feelings were at the time;
- an evaluation of the experience or event (what was good and bad about it);
- your analysis of the experience (what sense you can make of it).

It is always a good idea to make explicit use of a reflective model. For instance, Gibbs' reflective cycle (see Chapter 3) is a popular model that encourages a description of a past situation, analysis of feelings, evaluation of the experience, and an examination of what you would do if the situation arose again. You may use this model for your reflective essay, but you will have to use more analysis in each of its stages if you are writing at level 3 or Honours level. Another possible model is the framework for reflexive practice (Rolfe *et al.*, 2001). This framework is based on three questions: 'What?', 'So what?' and 'And now what?' that are supposed to stimulate reflection at different levels. The first question should start you reflecting upon the situation for you to be able to describe it. The second question encourages you to construct a personal theory about the situation and to learn from it. The third and, according to the developers of the framework, the most important stage should help you consider how you can improve the situation and the consequences of your own actions. Yet another model is Johns' (2004) model of structured reflection. This model can be used for general reflection on experience as well as for analysing more complex processes such as a critical incident, making it ideal for analysis at level 3 or Honours level.

Let us look at one concrete example of planning and structuring the body of the reflective essay following Gibbs' model. Notice how analysis permeates each of the body sections. Here is the question for the reflective essay, followed by the marking criteria:

> *How have your clinical knowledge and skills developed to help you meet the requirements for registering as a nurse?*

The marking criteria given for this essay are:

- work clearly presented, easy to read, free from spelling and grammar mistakes;

- shows ability to reflect on own knowledge and skills, identifying main issues and problems associated with professional practice;
- demonstrates ability to make a clear link between theory and practice;
- can make connections between requirements for registration and knowledge and skills developed;
- shows ability to integrate evidence-based support from the literature;
- demonstrates capacity for identifying future needs;
- accurately referenced following academic conventions (see Chapter 10).

Here is one possible way of planning and structuring the information in the body of the reflective essay in reference to the essay question and the

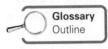
Glossary
Outline

marking criteria above. You have been given the **outline** for the introduction so that you can see the relationship between the body and the introduction:

- **Introduction**: introduce topic (what?): how can the requirements for registration be met; the focus (what exactly?): main requirements for registration: principles behind client-centred care, understanding of culture-sensitive practices, literacy and numeracy skills; signpost (how) reflecting upon experiences on course and on clinical placements.
- **Body section 1**: Topic: principles re client-centred care. Requirement for registration, how principles developed (literature), how theory informed clinical practice and vice versa (literature), what has been learnt from reflection (connection with experience), identification of future needs.
- **Body section 2**: Topic: culture-sensitive practices. Requirement for registration, how understanding developed (literature), how theory informed clinical practice and vice versa (literature), what has been learnt from reflection (connection with experience), identification of future needs.
- **Body section 3**: Topic: literacy. Requirement for registration, literacy development (literature), how theory informed clinical practice and vice versa (literature), what has been learnt from reflection (connection with experience), identification of future needs.
- **Body section 4**: Topic: numeracy. Requirement for registration, numeracy development (literature), how theory informed clinical practice and vice versa (literature), what has been learnt from

reflection (connection with experience), identification of future needs.

Notice how planning the essay following the organizing principle presented in the introduction (general-to-specific) has contributed to its structure. The paragraphs in the body develop the main issues identified in the focus of the introduction and have been developed in the way it was signposted in the introduction.

● Reflection and the conclusion of the essay

Conclusions serve the purpose of bringing the essay to a satisfactory end. This means that your conclusion should show the relationship between the different parts of the essay (see Chapter 1). The conclusion of a reflective essay will then:

- provide a summary of the issues explored in the body of the essay;
- remind the reader of the main purpose of the essay; and
- suggest an appropriate course of action in relation to the needs identified in the body of the essay.

The introduction and the body of the reflective essay presented in the previous section can be concluded by:

Activity 4.2

Read the following conclusion that has been written following the outline above. Has the conclusion been developed in an effective way? Be prepared to give reasons to support your answer.

Client-centred care is one of the basic principles that a nurse should learn to provide. It conceives of the client as a holistic individual. This principle should form the basis of both the theory and the practice of nursing care. To provide client-centred care, nurses should be able to recognize culture-sensitive practices and the way these are related to social cultures in general (Papalexandris, 2004). Societal characteristics are important sources of information for nurses to be able to make informed decisions in their daily practice. Informed decisions will obviously be the result of reflection on practice and respect for ethnicity, culture and differences.

Answers See suggested answers on page 193.

- summarizing main issues identified;
- drawing reader's attention to focus (principles behind client-centred care, understanding of culture-sensitive practices, literacy and numeracy skills); and
- identifying a course of action that links back to the needs identified in the body paragraphs.

Problem	Solution	Examples
The use of personal pronouns It may seem appropriate to use personal pronouns, especially 'I', to refer to personal experiences on placement. However, the use of personal pronouns may be distracting for the reader, drawing their attention to the writer rather than to the experience being analysed	**Change the focus of attention** Make the experience and what you have learnt from it the focus of your writing	☒ I will reflect upon my experience with a double-diagnosis patient during my clinical placement ☑ This essay will reflect on the writer's clinical experience with a double-diagnosis patient
The use of contracted forms Contracted forms (e.g. isn't, haven't, I'll, etc.) are representative of informal speech. Remember a reflective essay is a piece of formal writing	**Spell out all contractions** Use full words (is not, have not, I will, etc.) rather than contracted forms	☒ The patient wasn't prepared for the event as he hadn't been told about it ☑ The patient was not prepared for the event as he had not been told about it
The use of informal language Similarly, informal language is commonly used in other non-academic genres (e.g. personal letters)	**Use formal language** Formal language is careful and accurate language, characterized by formal vocabulary and impersonal structures	☒ I kind of know what it is but I can't really say much about postoperative pain, you know ☑ Postoperative pain is a difficult concept to define and requires a precise approach
Unsupported claims Unsupported claims are usually accepted in spoken genres and when you want to present or discuss your personal opinions	**Use references from the literature** In academic writing, every substantial claim that you make should be supported by some form of evidence (e.g. references from books, journal articles, etc.)	☒ Many have talked about the importance of communication in nursing for a long time ☑ The importance of communication in nursing has been at the centre of professional debates for many years (Atkinson, 1985; Smith, 1990; Orr, 2004)

Figure 4.1   Style problems in the reflective essay

● Grammar and English use

In this last section of the chapter we will analyse the style of the reflective essay. Figure 4.1 on the previous page shows some common problems and how to solve them, and for easy referencing, these problems are examined in the form of a trouble-shooting list. If you feel you need more detail on any of these topics, see the Glossary of Key Terms and the list of Further Readings and Resources at the end of the book.

Revising the objectives of this chapter

Tick those objectives you feel you have achieved and review those you have not yet managed to accomplish. Then complete the **Achievement Chart** at the back of the book.

In this chapter, you have learnt to:

☐ plan a reflective essay appropriately;

☐ identify an effective way of introducing reflective essays;

☐ recognize the structure of body paragraphs to support introductions;

☐ recognize ways of producing an effective conclusion;

☐ identify the style of the reflective essay.

5 How to Write a Care Critique

At the end of this chapter, you should be able to:

▶ define the care critique
▶ plan and organize the care critique effectively
▶ structure the main sections of the care critique
▶ provide effective conclusions and make sensible recommendations

Defining the care critique

In Chapter 2 we considered the basic elements of a care critique. In this chapter we examine how to structure and organize the care critique in more depth.

Before considering the organization and structure of a critique, let us explore words or phrases we associate with 'a critique'.

Pre-reading task: Re-read the section on the 'argumentative essay' in Chapter 2 before reading this chapter.

Activity 5.1

Put a tick (✔) next to the words or phrases you consider related to 'a critique' and a cross (✘) next to those which you think are not related. Then draw arrows to join the central balloon with those you have ticked.

Analytical thinking

Critical reading

Argumentative

A CRITIQUE

Likes & dislikes

Descriptive

Evaluative

Answers See suggested answers on page 194.

77

A critique requires presenting a balanced evaluation of what is being considered. For this, you will need all the reflective skills examined in Chapter 3. Thus, words such as *analytical thinking* and *evaluative* are closely associated with a critique.

Activity 5.2

Considering what you have learnt in Chapter 2 and your choices in Activity 5.1, how would you define a 'care critique'?

_____

_____

_____

_____

_____

_____

_____

How does your definition compare with the one given below?

> *A care critique is a* **systematic**, **critical** *and* **impersonal** *analysis of the care provided that discusses its* **validity** *and evaluates its* **worth**.

The words in bold are central to this definition of a care critique and merit further comment. Let us start with the first three: **systematic**, **critical** and **impersonal**.

'Systematic' refers to doing something in a coherent, thorough and principled way over a given period of time. Supposing you want to examine systematically the care that patients who have had a minor accident receive after being discharged from hospital. You will first have to decide what is understood by 'care' and 'minor accident'. You will also need to examine this care over a given period of time, and focus on a patient who meets the criteria specified. Put together, these three things represent examining the care in a systematic way.

'Critical', as you examined in Chapter 3, is related to being able to:

- identify the position or view of the people involved in providing and receiving the care (i.e. what the professionals who provide the care think about it, and what the patients who receive the care think about it);
- evaluate the reasons for providing the care and whether they were valid or not; and
- present a given point of view (probably based on the reasons or views of the professionals and the patients).

'Impersonal' refers to both your position on what you are analysing (not personally involved or attached) and the language that you use to represent the object of your analysis (e.g. using impersonal language and structures).

The other two words '**validity**' and '**worth**' are closely connected with the verb 'to evaluate'. As we saw in Chapter 1, this means to determine the significance of something, usually by careful appraisal and study. In this sense, for your readers to realize the significance of the care, you will have to provide them with the positive and negative aspects of the care given. Based on the negative aspects you examined, you will have to then provide some recommendations as discussed later in the chapter.

To recap, a care critique is a systematic analysis of the care given to a patient. It is not a subjective recount of the facts, but an objective evaluation of the care with recommendations for better practice.

Planning and organizing the critique

Now that we have defined a care critique so we know what it **is**, let us deal with what it **does**. A care critique has four essential aims. It should:

- identify and outline a well-defined problem or issue;
- analyse issues in the care and data that can be used as evidence;
- provide a solution or solutions to the problem; and
- demonstrate what action needs to be taken if necessary.

As you can see there are five main **verbs** that indicate the purpose of a care critique, so let us analyse these verbs more closely:

- identify: recognize something so that you can say **who/what** it is;
- outline: give a brief description of the **main facts** or **points**;
- analyse: examine the nature or structure of something in order to provide **a better understanding** or an **explanation** of it;

- provide: make something available in a way that **can be used** or **put into practice**;
- demonstrate: show something clearly, providing **support**, **proof** or **evidence**.

We need to remember something very important here – the basis for our analysis is *identifying*. If we don't identify the problem or an issue, none of the rest is possible. It is also important that we *outline* the problem for which the care was provided, rather than describe it in detail as would be done in a case study. Remember that the focus of the critique is the care provided and not the problem itself. The problem serves as background information to the care and is usually outlined in the first part of the body of the critique.

Once you have identified and briefly described the problem or issue, it is time for you to focus on the central aims of the care critique: analyse the issues, provide solutions and recommend a course of action.

Here is a generic structure you could use to plan and organize your care critiques. Whenever you have to write a care critique, you can use the lines provided to jot down your own ideas about the contents.

Note that the 'body' section contains three issues. This is because in a typical 2,000-word critique, you can only cover three or four related issues with a certain depth. In longer pieces you could have more. However, you will always have to strike a balance between width and depth. Too many issues will require more words and you will be unable to deal with them in appropriate depth.

I Introduction

Topic: (Go back to the care critique question.)

_____

Focus: (Issues you want to raise in connection with the care; connect issues with the learning outcomes of the module.)

_____

Aims: (What will your critique specifically do? How will it do it?)

_____

II Body

Identify and outline the problem: (A brief description of the patient, the context, the need for care and what was done.)

_____

Issue 1: (Identify issue and the sources you will use as support or evidence.)

_____

Issue 2: (Identify issue and the sources you will use as support or evidence.)

_____

Issue 3: (Identify issue and the sources you will use as support or evidence.)

_____

III Conclusion

Summarize main points:

_____

Revisit your focus:

_____

Discuss validity/worth of care:

_____

Make recommendations: (To resolve problems/issues addressed in body.)

_____

● Structuring the care critique

Once you have finished planning the contents of the care critique, you will need to structure its information.

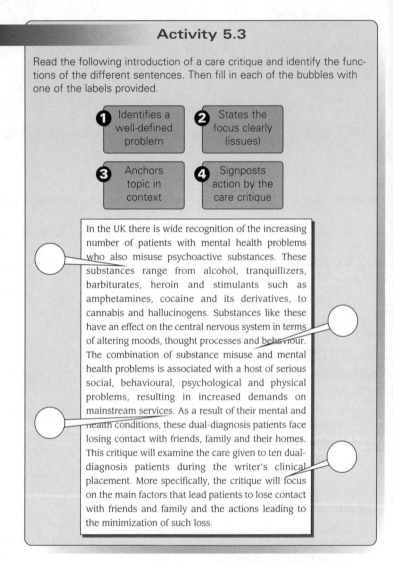

Activity 5.3

Read the following introduction of a care critique and identify the functions of the different sentences. Then fill in each of the bubbles with one of the labels provided.

1 Identifies a well-defined problem

2 States the focus clearly (issues)

3 Anchors topic in context

4 Signposts action by the care critique

In the UK there is wide recognition of the increasing number of patients with mental health problems who also misuse psychoactive substances. These substances range from alcohol, tranquillizers, barbiturates, heroin and stimulants such as amphetamines, cocaine and its derivatives, to cannabis and hallucinogens. Substances like these have an effect on the central nervous system in terms of altering moods, thought processes and behaviour. The combination of substance misuse and mental health problems is associated with a host of serious social, behavioural, psychological and physical problems, resulting in increased demands on mainstream services. As a result of their mental and health conditions, these dual-diagnosis patients face losing contact with friends, family and their homes. This critique will examine the care given to ten dual-diagnosis patients during the writer's clinical placement. More specifically, the critique will focus on the main factors that lead patients to lose contact with friends and family and the actions leading to the minimization of such loss.

Answers See suggested answers on page 194.

The main sentences in this introduction serve very specific functions (or moves) that indicate to the reader the way the information is going to be dealt with in the rest of the text. As you probably realized in Activity 5.3,

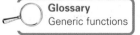

Glossary
Generic functions

there are **generic functions** that readers will expect to find in your introduction:

- locating the topic in the general context of the discussion;
- identifying a well-defined problem and its main issues;
- stating the focus of the critique;
- signposting what the care critique will do.

As you saw in the generic structure presented above, the body of your care critique will then develop the issues you have identified in the introduction. The basic functions of the body of a critique are to:

- present an objective summary of the care;
- identify a problem or problems with the care;
- establish the main issues associated with the problem;
- critically discuss these issues using research-based evidence (e.g. references); and
- demonstrate what it is appropriate to do about the identified problem and its associated issues.

● Concluding and making recommendations

The last section of the care critique is the **conclusion** (see also Chapter 1) and **recommendations**. This section of the critique should show three moves:

- restate the identification of the problem;
- summarize the main issues;
- recommend a course of action that will improve the care critiqued.

To write conclusions that wrap up the contents of the care critique in a satisfactory manner, you should take the following into account:

- when restating the problem, focus on why this problem is **relevant** in the context of the care;
- when summarizing the main issues, state their **significance** in relation to the problem critiqued;
- when making recommendations revisit the **weaknesses** of the care.

Activity 5.4

Read the following example of a conclusion of a critique that examines the care provided to a woman in the third stage of labour. Considering what you have learnt about conclusions so far, how effective do you think this conclusion is? Give reasons for your answer.

This care critique has analysed the midwifery care given to Mrs M, during the third stage of labour. The period following delivery of a baby should be a time of relief and joy for all those involved. However, this period holds great potential dangers for the mother. Post partum haemorrhage (PPH) has been identified as one of the main complications of the third stage which accounts for the highest maternal mortality and morbidity. As demonstrated in this care, there is compelling evidence that lends support to the benefits of active management of the third stage as it decreases complications and morbidity, especially in high-risk cases. There is strong advocacy for prophylactic syntocinon administration during delivery of the baby and other medications commonly used in the active management of third stage of labour as well as for CCT with counter-traction when the uterus is well-contracted. There is also strong support for planning in advance and active management.

Answers See suggested answers on page 195.

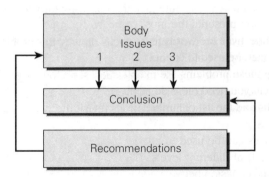

Figure 5.1   The relationship between conclusion and recommendations

The recommendations that you make have to be connected with the body and the conclusion of the care critique. Recommendations should establish a **logical relationship** with the issues addressed in the body of the critique and should **sensibly result** from the conclusion that you have presented. Figure 5.1 represents this connection.

The following text illustrates the type of recommendations that you could make to go with the conclusion presented in Activity 5.4 above.

Activity 5.5

How appropriate would you say the recommendations made here are?

Midwives must be able to identify women at high risk, and make plans for emergency management so as to be prepared to deal with complications in a timely and systematic manner. It is recommended that clear and effective guidelines be provided to all midwives as well as training incorporated to support midwives in making the best possible decisions.

Answers See suggested answers on page 195.

Table 5.1 presents a checklist of things that you should consider after you have finished writing your care critique. Remember to plan some action to improve those aspects of the critique to which you have given a negative answer. Add new questions to the checklist as you use it more regularly.

● Grammar and English use

This last section presents the most common connectives used in academic writing. Connectives are words (e.g. 'and', 'but', 'so') or phrases (e.g. 'on the one hand') that are used to connect ideas, sentences or longer texts. For easy referencing, these problems are examined in the form of a trouble-shooting list. If you feel you need more detail on any of these topics, see the Glossary of Key Terms and the list of Further Readings and Resources at the end of the book.

Connectives can be used to provide cohesion (sticking together) to texts (see Chapter 1) at different levels. They can be used (see Table 5.2 on page 87) to provide cohesion between ideas in (1) the same sentence, (2) different sentences, and (3) longer pieces of writing, as the following texts illustrate:

Questions	Yes/No	Action if 'no'
1 Have you presented the **introduction** clearly, indicating **topic**, **focus** and **comment**?		
2 Have you **structured** the body of your critique **effectively** (e.g. developing one issue in each section)?		
3 Have you presented an **objective summary** of the care provided?		
4 Have you clearly **identified the problems** with the care and their associated issues?		
5 Have you presented the **issues** in the body of your critique in a **balanced** and **comprehensive** manner?		
6 Have you supported these issues by **specific examples** from clinical placement and **evidence** from the literature?		
7 Have you demonstrated what would be **appropriate to do** about the identified problem?		
8 Have you shown why this problem is **relevant** in the context of the care?		
9 Have you stated the **significance of the issues** explored in relation to the problem critiqued?		
10 Have you **recommended a course of action** that will improve the weaknesses of the care critiqued?		

Table 5.1 Checklist for the care critique

To	You can use	For example
add an idea	and, also, as well as, furthermore, in addition, next, another, other ...	**Another example** of the complex relationship between ...
add an opposing idea	but, however, on the other hand, in contrast, although, nevertheless, on the contrary, conversely ...	**On the other hand**, this attitude has attracted a great deal of opposition from ...
add a similar idea	similarly, likewise, also, as, once again ...	**Also**, we have to consider how many other possibilities lie ...
give an example/ examples	for example, for instance, as follows ...	We could say, **for instance**, that these reasons have not been well ...
express exceptions, or reservation	even though, still, yet, nevertheless, ...	They have been widely researched. **Yet** the results provided by most studies ...
give an alternative	in other words, or rather, alternatively, ...	**In other words**, we can go on like this for ever and ever.
identify a cause	for, because, since, as, ...	**Because** they didn't have all the necessary people in their team, they couldn't finish the project in time.
give an effect	therefore, thus, hence, consequently, as a result, so, ...	They couldn't finish the project in time, **so** part of their fees ...
list ideas in time order or order of importance	first, second, third, etc. then, next, finally, ...	**First**, the essay will present an overview of ...
mark a transition	now, as far as X is concerned, with regards to, as for, ...	**As far as time is concerned**, I would like to make the following observations.
make a generalization	in general, on the whole, in most cases, usually, frequently, mainly, ...	**On the whole**, these cases show that most patients would prefer ...
highlight	in particular, especially, particularly, ...	**In particular**, this section of the dissertation will focus on ...
give a summary, or conclusion	in summary, to conclude, in short,	**In short**, these are the three main issues that ...

Table 5.2   The use of connectives

1 The patient was in cardiac arrest **and** was assisted by an automated defibrillator.
2 This kind of support has proved very effective in helping pregnant smokers cope with cravings. **On the other hand**, it has not had lasting effects after childbirth.
3 Many arguments have been advanced in favour of the benefits of returning a patient with a stroke to the open plan unit (Brown, 1999; Thompson, 2004; Willis, 2002). **These** include the positive support reported by the patients and the quality of the follow-up care. **However**, the advantages of allowing patients with a stroke to stay in the same room have not been fully examined (Allen, 2001).

Revising the objectives of this chapter

Tick those objectives you feel you have achieved and review those you have not yet managed to accomplish. Then complete the **Achievement Chart** at the back of the book.

In this chapter, you have learnt to:

☐ Define the care critique

☐ Plan and organize the care critique effectively

☐ Structure the main sections of the care critique

☐ Provide effective conclusions and make sensible recommendations

6 How to Write an Argument

At the end of this chapter, you should be able to:

▶ recognize the difference between opinion and argumentation
▶ identify the strength of an argument
▶ structure arguments effectively
▶ identify main language items used in argumentative writing

Pre-reading task: Re-read the section on the 'argumentative essay' in Chapter 2 before reading this chapter.

● Evaluating claims

Read the following two statements. Which states an opinion? Which one presents an argument?

> Many professionals would now agree that the results of research in midwifery care are inconclusive and even contradictory.
> **A**

> Previous studies have shown that results of midwifery care research are inconclusive and sometimes contradictory (Kirkham, 2002; Powell Kennedy and Shannon, 2004; Raisler, 2000). However, recent research has demonstrated that …
> **B**

Whereas **claim** A sounds very formal and authoritative, it is nonetheless stating an opinion. There is no evidence that supports the claim, so we can say claim A simply states what the speaker or writer assumes to be true. Statement B, on the other hand, is a statement of a fact supported by evidence. As you read in Chapter 2, opinion claims do not necessarily have to be supported by evidence. You can say 'nursing is a difficult profession' and do not need to provide evidence of that. However, evidence is important in argumentation as it is the basis upon which your argument will rest. If you express an opinion, there is then no argument, unless your opinion is challenged and you need to support it using evidence. Only then will you have an argument.

🔍 **Glossary**
Claim

There are some questions that you can use to check whether the claim you are reading or making is a statement of opinion or an argument. Consider:

- Can you identify a clearly defined position taken on the topic?
- Have alternative positions been provided?
- Is there a call to action (e.g. recommendation)?

If two answers to these questions are negative, then you have an opinion in front of you. Use the questions to check example A above, for instance. There is no *clearly* identified position; there is only a vaguely stated idea. Similarly, no alternative positions have been provided and no action has been called.

Here is another list of questions. You can use these to challenge an argument. These questions should help you measure the strength of a claim, and thus also enable you to discern opinions from arguments:

- Does the claim reflect the writer's belief? If so, is the belief supported by other evidence-based arguments?
- Does the claim present evidence that both supports and contradicts it?
- How are the claim and the evidence related? Closely or only indirectly?

Apart from these questions, you may also think of the logic of argumentation in order to evaluate claims. What is the logic of an argument? Any **claims** will start with what the writer thinks or believes to be true. But, this is an opinion. To make this claim a fact, they will need to provide **evidence**. Based on this, writers can then present their **conclusion** or conclusions about the fact or facts they have expressed. Now, you must make sure that their conclusions result from both the evidence and the claims they have made. The relationship between these three elements in the logic of arguments was illustrated in Figure 2.3 in Chapter 2.

Remember the following:

- **Analyse the thesis**: if the starting claim (thesis) is faulty, the whole argument is. Sometimes the thesis needs to be **toned down** as it does not always apply. For instance, the thesis may claim that 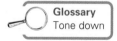 a certain situation applies to (all) women in labour, but the evidence exemplifies only primagravida women. In this case the thesis needs toning down.

  Glossary
  Tone down

- **Analyse the relationship** between the presupposition, the supporting evidence and the conclusion. Watch out for particular instances and general claims, and inconsistencies in the relationship between the three.

● **Examine the conclusion**: the conclusion must logically develop from the thesis and the supporting evidence. Sometimes the claims are acceptable, but the conclusion drawn from them is not.

Activity 6.1

Analyse the following statements and decide whether they are claims stating opinions (OP) or facts (FA). Be prepared to support your choices.

1 It has, for example, been suggested that whereas health promotion programmes at the national level have successfully met their targets, at more local levels similar programmes have failed to accommodate the needs of a growing population.

2 Previous studies have strongly supported the initiative of helping pregnant women stop smoking. However, some of these studies have produced inconclusive evidence in relation to the efficacy of support programmes for pregnant smokers (e.g. Kelley *et al.*, 2001; Melvin *et al.*, 2000; Melvin & Gaffney, 2004).

3 We would argue that there is an ever-growing need for needs analysis exercises to determine the real needs of local populations in relation to midwifery health promotion.

4 Management of diabetes is improved if appropriately trained practice nurses are involved.

Answers See suggested answers on page 195.

● **The strength of an argument**

A strong argument will not only support its claims by providing evidence-based examples or support, but will incorporate and challenge opposing arguments, showing their weaknesses and how these could be solved.

One way in which you can work with opposing arguments is by analysing them *vis-à-vis* your own thesis. It is a good idea to start by making a list of the strengths and the weaknesses of the opposing arguments, so that they can be compared with the strengths and weaknesses of your own arguments.

Table 6.1 illustrates how the comparison between two opposing arguments can be charted on a table. This will not only help you see how the two arguments compare, but also how you can use them to structure your texts as we shall discuss in the next section.

Topic: The role of technology in the intensive care unit (ICU)			
Argument A: technological approach to ICU (e.g. Ray, 1987; Benner et al., 1992)		**Argument B**: techno-ethico-human approach to ICU (Walters, 1995; Alasad, 2002)	
Strengths	*Weaknesses*	*Strengths*	*Weaknesses*
S.1 The importance of technical aspects. **S.2** The importance that to ICU nurses give care in this context.	**W.1** The effects of technology on ICU nurses have been ignored. **W.2** ICU nurses have been seen as technical agents.	**S.1** Focuses on the effects that technology can have on critical care nurses. **S.2** Follows a techno-ethico-human caring model.	**W.1** Deemphasizes the importance of technical skills in nurses.

Table 6.1 Argument comparison table

Table 6.1 shows how the weaknesses of one argument can be related to the strengths of the other. For example, the first weakness of argument A (the effects of technology on ICU nurses has been ignored) can be contrasted with the first strength of argument B (focuses on the effects that technology can have on critical care nurses). If you had to write an argument using these claims, you could then produce something like

> *The role of technology in the intensive care unit (ICU) has been the focus of a debate which has intensified in the last decade (Ray, 1987; Benner et al., 1992; Walters, 1995; Alasad, 2002). Some of these studies have followed a technological approach to issues relating to the ICU. They have mainly emphasized the importance of the technical aspects of the ICU and of the significance given to the care by critical care nurses (e.g. Ray, 1987; Benner et al., 1992). However, they have ignored the effects of technology on ICU nurses and have shown a tendency to see critical care nurses as technical agents. This study advocates a change of emphasis from technology to ethics, following what has been recognized as a techno-ethico-human model of care (Walters, 1995; Alasad, 2002).*

Activity 6.2

Based on the information in the following text, complete the argument comparison table below.

An essential first step in pressure ulcers prevention is the identification of those patients who are truly at risk. Since the early 1960s a variety of risk assessment scales (RAS) has been developed with over 20 such instruments currently described in the world-wide literature (Torra I Bou, 1998). These scales assign numerical values to various patient traits (such as their level of mobility) with a total score generated from the sum of these values. Considerable attention has been given to comparison of different scales based upon statistical constructs such as their sensitivity and specificity (Cullum *et al.*, 1995; Anthony *et al.*, 2000). However, such activity is subject to a major limitation; when risk has been identified preventive interventions are initiated, and so the 'true' sensitivity of any RAS cannot be measured. (Papanikolaou *et al.*, 2002: 187–8)

Topic: Risk assessment scales for preventing pressure ulcers

Argument A (*For*):	**Argument B** (*Against*):
Strengths	*Weaknesses*

Answers See suggested answers on page 196.

● The structure of argumentation

As we have examined in previous chapters, planning is a central activity in writing, and this also applies to writing arguments. Planning will help focus your ideas and make sure they are presented clearly and logically. The following guide will help you think through the planning process and structure your work clearly when writing argumentative texts (see also Table 2.3 in Chapter 2).

- **Introduction**: What is the topic of your argumentative essay? What is its aim? What claim(s) do you want to make in it?
- **Main points**: What reasons will you give to justify your claim(s)? What reasons will you give to support your conclusions?
- **Supporting statements**: Apart from including your supporting points, what other points that contradict or place doubt on the argument will you discuss? How will you balance your statements?
- **Summary**: How will you review your discussion? What points will you highlight? How will you highlight them?
- **Conclusion**: How will you call the reader's attention to the main issues identified in your introduction? Will you include a brief discussion of alternatives for the future? How will you examine implications of the conclusions? Will you make recommendations based on the conclusions you presented?

Activity 6.3

Analyse the following text and decide how you could turn it into an argumentative text.

Many professionals would now agree that the results of research in midwifery care are inconclusive and sometimes even contradictory. It has, for example, been suggested that whereas health promotion programmes at the national level have successfully met their targets, at more local levels similar programmes have failed to accommodate the needs of a growing population.

Answers See suggested answers on page 196.

Structurally an argumentative text should include these four elements:

- A statement of the topic (1);
- Argument or arguments that contradict the thesis (2);
- A transitional marker marking a contradiction (3);
- Statement of the thesis (4).

The structure and organization of these elements in a text are illustrated in the following short text by Jenkins and Elliot (2004: 623):

Occupatinal stress in the nursing profession has been the
focus of much research over the last 20 years (Gray-Toft &
Anderson, 1981; Packard & Motowidlo, 1987; Dewe, 1989;
Foxall *et al.*, 1990; Tyler & Ellison, 1994; Brown & Edelmann,
2000). However, Dunn and Ritter (1995) have noted that
relatively few studies have investigated mental health nurses.
Although many of the pressures faced by this group are
similar to those reported by staff in other nursing specialities
(Riding & Wheeler, 1995), a number of demands relate
specifically to mental health settings. These include the often
intense nature of nurse–patient interaction (Cronin-Stubbs &
Brophy, 1985) and the confrontation of difficult and
challenging behaviours on a regular basis (Sullivan, 1993).

Activity 6.4

Analyse the following texts and decide how these four elements have
been organized.

Text 1

The debate surrounding evidence-based practice and the implementation of research-based knowledge in practice is well rehearsed.
Some of the key issues discussed have been perceived as barriers
to the implementation of knowledge, with Funk *et al.* (1991) developing a 'barriers to research utilisation' questionnaire that has been
widely adopted in the National Health Service (Retsas, 2000; Closs
et al., 2000; Parahoo, 2000). However, these barriers have been
mostly framed as individual responsibility – the lack of skill in
research critique, the lack of interest in accessing the written knowledge base, the lack of compliance with the evidence (Kaluzny *et al.*,
1995; French, 1996). (Clarke & Wilcockson, 2002: 397)

Text 2

While in recent years there has been an increase in the number of
studies examining occupational stress among community mental
health nurses (Harper & Minghella, 1997; McLeod, 1997; Coffey,
1999; Drake & Brumblecombe, 1999; Burnard *et al.*, 2000), the
experiences of staff in acute inpatient settings, providing 24-hour
care for people with serious mental illness, have received less
attention. An investigation of acute mental health nursing commissioned for the United Kingdom's (UK) Department of Health (Higgins
et al., 1997) has highlighted the need for further research in this
area. (Jenkins & Elliot, 2004: 623)

Answers See suggested answers on page 196.

Table 6.2 presents a checklist of things that you should consider after you have finished writing your argumentative essays. Remember to plan an action to take if your answer to any of the questions has been negative. As you use the checklist more regularly, add new questions to it so that it becomes more relevant to your needs as a writer.

Questions	Yes/No	Action if 'no'
1 Have you clearly stated the topic of your argument, its aim(s) and your claims in the **introduction**?		
2 Have you given **reasons** to justify your claims and **support** your conclusions?		
3 Have you presented a **balanced consideration** of opposing arguments?		
4 Have you used **evidence** to support your claims as well as evidence that supports opposing claims?		
5 Have you briefly **summarized** the claims made, highlighting the main issues or points discussed?		
6 Have you **concluded** in a satisfactory manner, examining implications and making recommendations (if necessary)?		
7 . . .		

Table 6.2   Checklist for the argumentative essay

● The language of arguments

The language of arguments is simple, straightforward and forceful, rather than poetic or fanciful. One of the main linguistic features of argumentative essays is transitional words or connectives (see Chapters 1 and 5), because we need to keep arguments either tightly together as when we want to high-light similarities, or widely apart as when we want to emphasize how they differ.

Another common feature in arguments is the use of words that indicate the position of the writers in relation to the argument. This relates to writer stance, as explored in Chapter 3. To indicate this relation, writers have a set of linguistic tools at their disposal, some of which are:

- Modal verbs: e.g. 'may', 'can', 'could' to indicate various degrees of possibility; 'would', 'should', and 'will' for various degrees of prob-ability; and 'must', 'have to', and 'ought to' to express degrees of certainty;
- Adverbials: e.g. 'possibly', 'probably', 'certainly';
- Connectives: e.g. 'in as much as', 'for the reason that', 'conse-quently';
- Verbal phrases: e.g. 'it follows that', 'it may be inferred that', 'it may be concluded that'.

● Grammar and English use

In this last section of the chapter you will find some suggestions about how to deal with grammar and language-use problems that many students expe-rience when writing argumentative texts. More specifically, this section deals with the language of argumentation. If you need more detail on any of these topics, see the Glossary of Key Terms and the list of Further Readings and Resources at the end of the book.

Modal verbs

Modal verbs are special verbs that indicate 'the way or mode' in which something is done or said. In sentence (1) the modal verb 'will' does not indi-cate future but the way the speaker sees the possibility of something happen-ing. In sentence (2) the speaker appears less certain and therefore chooses to decrease the level of certainty by using 'may'.

1 The patient *will* find it difficult to adjust herself to her new lifestyle.
2 The patient *may* find it difficult to adjust herself to her new lifestyle.

Table 6.3 on page 99 shows you the most frequent uses of common modal verbs, followed by some examples.

Activity 6.5

Read these two versions of the same text: version 1 is merely descriptive and version 2 is argumentative. Underline those features of language that have helped to make the second version argumentative.

Version 1

The differences seen are not explainable by disappointment with the care-giver assignment. Staniszewska and Ahmed (1999) point out that patients' expectations are influenced by their awareness of what they realistically expect. Evaluation of a service is also influenced by beliefs about the duty the service owes the client and whether or not there were circumstances outside the service's control that affected the care (Williams *et al.*, 1998). If expectations are a determinant of satisfaction with care, there is then less difference between the satisfaction scores of the two groups since women have different expectations for doctors than they do for midwives. (Adapted from: Harvey *et al.*, 2002: 266)

Version 2

It is possible, however, that the differences seen are not entirely explainable by disappointment with the care-giver assignment. Staniszewska and Ahmed (1999) point out that patients' expectations are influenced by their awareness of what they might realistically expect. Evaluation of a service is also influenced by beliefs about the duty the service owes the client and whether or not there were circumstances outside the service's control that affected the care (Williams *et al.*, 1998). If expectations are a determinant of satisfaction with care, it is possible that there would have been less difference between the satisfaction scores of the two groups since women have different expectations for doctors than they do for midwives. (Harvey *et al.*, 2002: 266)

Answers See suggested answers on page 197.

As you can see from the table, there are various possibilities to express a similar meaning, indicated by the numbers in brackets. For example, there are at least four different ways of expressing possibility, which can be put on a cline to indicate different degrees, as indicated below.

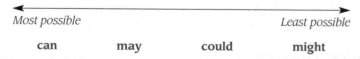

Most possible   *Least possible*

can   **may**   **could**   **might**

Put simply, the difference in meaning between sentences (3)–(6) (p. 100) is only one of the degree of possibility.

Modal verb	Meaning 1	Meaning 2
Can	*Ability* She **can** speak many languages, which has helped her deal with her diverse patients.	*Possibility* (1) The results of this study **can** make a real impact on the professional practice of midwives.
Could	*Possibility* (2) You **could** spend the rest of your free time revising for your exams tomorrow.	*Suggestion* These results **could** indicate progress can be a slippery concept.
Have to	*Certainty* (1) That **has to** be the right dose for a patient in his condition.	*Obligation* (1) You **have to** follow the doctor's orders if you want to be discharged from hospital soon.
May	*Possibility* (3) Under these psychiatric conditions, the patient **may** temporarily lose control over his or her actions.	*Permission* Patients **may** not bring their own personal belongings with them unless they are told to do so.
Might	*Possibility* (4) Under his psychiatric conditions, the patient **might** temporarily lose control over his or her actions.	*Suggestion* You **might** not want to be alone when you come to collect the results of the test.
Must	*Certainty* (2) That **must** have been the best possible way of doing it.	*Obligation* (2) You **must** bring with you a proof of identity and your medical record number.
Shall	*Inevitability* The drug **shall** react in a matter of seconds.	*Promise* I **shall** make the shift arrangements for tomorrow.
Should	*Recommendation* They **should** have followed the directions as they were indicated.	*Assumption* They **should** be here by now.

Table 6.3   The use of modal verbs

3 The results of this study **can** make a real impact on the professional practice of midwives.

4 The results of this study **may** make a real impact on the professional practice of midwives.

5 The results of this study **could** make a real impact on the professional practice of midwives.

6 The results of this study **might** make a real impact on the professional practice of midwives.

Adverbials

Adverbials can also be used to indicate the writer's stance in relation to the claims made. Again, we could say that the difference between sentences (7) and (8) is one of degree:

7 The patient has made a speedy recovery.

8 The patient has **certainly** made a speedy recovery.

Other adverbials that indicate the writer's stance include: possibly, probably, certainly, definitely, inevitably, forcefully, successfully, unfortunately.

Verbal phrases

Verbal phrases that contain verbs such as 'seem', 'appear', 'look', or adverbials like the ones described above can also be used to indicate stance. Sentences (10)–(12) show not only the degree of certainty of the writer, but also the writer's stance in term of the claims being made.

10 Considering the results, **it may be concluded that** the tests have failed.

11 Considering the results, **it seems that** the tests have failed.

12 Considering the results, the tests **have failed**.

Revising the objectives of this chapter

Tick those objectives you feel you have achieved and review those you have not yet managed to accomplish. Then, complete the **Achievement Chart** at the back of the book.

In this chapter, you have learnt to:

☐ recognize the difference between opinion and argumentation

☐ identify the strength of an argument

☐ structure arguments effectively

☐ identify main language items used in argumentative writing

7 How to Write Other Genres

At the end of this chapter, you should be able to:

▶ write actions plans
▶ write care plans
▶ prepare, write and choose an appropriate format for portfolios
▶ produce reports
▶ identify effective ways of producing dissertation proposals
▶ plan to start writing your dissertation

Other common genres

In this chapter you will explore other common genres in nursing and midwifery – action and care plans, portfolios, reports and research proposals.

The chapter opens with an examination of what action plans are and what information you will need to complete them. It then moves on to describe care plans and examines the type of information and language that you use to complete them. Next, you will analyse portfolios. The section on portfolios provides you with a fairly comprehensive coverage of the topic: what portfolios are, what they contain, how they can be formatted and how they are normally assessed.

In the last part of the chapter you will deal with reports and with the research proposal. In the research proposal section you will find information about how to prepare and present a proposal, together with tips on what to include in each section and the appropriate style to use. Finally, you will find tips on how to get organized to write your undergraduate dissertation.

How to write action plans

Students often ask whether action plans are the same as 'to-do' lists. They do share some similarities, but they are not the same. To-do lists enumerate all the tasks that you need to carry out; they are useful reminders of what you have to do. They can include a priority ranking – you can rank each of the tasks as 'high priority', 'medium priority' or 'low priority'. Table 7.1 shows you what a to-do list looks like.

Action plans, on the other hand, do not only lay out the task you will concentrate on, but they also include a detailed description of the steps to be taken to successfully perform the task. Action plans also include challenges you might face in carrying out the tasks and strategies you can use to face

Task	Priority (H = high, M = medium, L = low)
1 Read chapters 5 & 6 in Atkinson's book for exam.	H
2 Return books to library before end of next week.	M
3 Email John & Marcia about a get-together after exams.	L

Table 7.1 A to-do list with priority ranking

those challenges. It is important that you give the task at hand a deadline for completion.

The information you enter in an action plan will help you monitor and assess your progress and record any changes that have been made in the process of getting things done. Action plans can be used on their own or they can be part of other documents such as your personal development plan or your portfolio (see later in the chapter). Table 7.2 illustrates an action plan for a very simple task: read two book chapters as preparation for an exam. Although you may not need a detailed action plan for simple tasks such as this, it is always a good idea to start with laying out simple tasks. As you get more practice, you will see that you don't need so many details and that your language in describing tasks, challenges and strategies becomes simpler and simpler.

The language and style of action plans is simple and straightforward. As illustrated in Table 7.2, you don't need to use complete sentences – notes will do. You will need different tenses for the different sections of an action plan; infinitives or the simple present tense are used to provide a short description of the task, the simple future to describe challenges and strategies, the present perfect tense to record progress and the simple past to indicate the completion of the task, though a simple date indicating when the task was completed would do.

● How to write care plans

What are care plans? Care plans are documents that provide a detailed description of the plan of care to be provided to a patient. Traditionally, care plans have been regarded to be the sole domain of nurses, but with the increase in the involvement of interdisciplinary teams in the care of patients, this should no longer be the case. For care plans to be effective, their design and implementation should engage not only nurses, but all the professionals who are involved in providing care to the patient.

Care-plan documents will normally include:

- The patient's name, his/her medical record number and his/her room number;
- Date and description of patient's needs and problems;
- nursing diagnoses (though this will depend on your work setting);
- goal-setting;
- interventions needed to achieve the goals;
- assessment of progress;
- re-evaluation of care plan.

What steps are followed in designing care plans? Your work setting may have an established protocol for care plans or may just have general guidelines, but most care plans will start by evaluating the patient's needs. This is referred to as the **first step**, and normally involves assessing the patient on admission.

The **second step** requires drawing up a problem list. Again, depending on your work setting, this may just mean a list of medical diagnoses but it could be more complicated protocols.

The **third step** is closely related to the second. Here you use information that comes from asking questions such as 'how can this be solved/improved?' for each of the problems on your list, followed by setting a goal to improve the problem. It is important to remember that each of the goals that you set should be SMART (Specific, Measurable, Attainable, Realistic and Time-orientated).

The **fourth step** will describe the actions or interventions needed to achieve each goal, while the **fifth step** assesses the progress made by the patient and re-evaluates the care plan to adjust it to the patient's changed needs. Figure 7.1 shows you the relationship of the five steps.

How are care plans written? What language is used and what tenses are required? The different parts of the care plan will require different language and tenses:

- **Description of problem/need**: Give a general label to the problem (e.g. communication), followed by a short description (e.g. has difficulty understanding what is being said). This is mainly

Task	Steps	Challenges (CH)/Strategies (ST)	Progress	Completion
1 Read chapter 5 (Atkinson) for exam in 2 wks.	1.1 Borrow book from library.	May not find available copy at library. (CH) Will have to borrow copy from another student & photocopy. (ST) Who will you call?	Done. There was a copy in library.	Day 1
	1.2 Read chapter 5 through.	Interruptions by flat mates. (CH) Study at library. (ST)	Finished reading	Day 1
	1.3 Underline main ideas.	May not find them easily. (CH) Photocopy & colour-code. (ST)	Done	Day 1
	1.4 Summarize main ideas.	Put ideas coded in same colour together. (ST)	Done	Day 1
	1.5 Read and write summary in own words.	Difficult to paraphrase, find synonymous expressions. (CH) Use dictionary/thesaurus. (ST)	Will tomorrow/ Done on day 2	Day 2
2. Read chapter 6 (Atkinson) for exam in 2 wks.	2.1 Read chapter 6 through.	Interruptions by flat mates. (CH) Study at library. (ST)	Finished reading	Day 2
	2.2 Underline main ideas.	May not find them easily. (CH) Photocopy & colour-code. (ST)	Done	Day 2
	2.3 Summarize main ideas.	Put ideas coded in same colour together. (ST)	Done	Day 2
	2.4 Read and write summary in own words.	Difficult to paraphrase, find synonymous expressions. (CH) Use dictionary/thesaurus (ST)	Done	Day 2

Table 7.2 Action plan for exam preparation

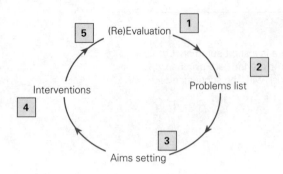

Figure 7.1 Steps in care planning

expressed in a present tense (the present perfect may also be used). You don't normally need subjects and there is a tendency not to use **articles** (the, a, etc.). For example, (*patient*) **has** (simple

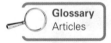

present) *knowledge deficit regarding transmission, complications and treatment of Chlamydia*, or *patient* **has been diagnosed** (present perfect) *with breast cancer*.

- **Goal-setting**: state the goal in simple terms, followed by the deadline expressed in days or months (use 'will' and verbal phrases such as 'be able to') as for example, *resident with a stroke will be able to communicate his basic needs in 2 months*. Avoid expressing two or more goals together. This would make it difficult for you to evaluate progress on each. The patient may make good progress towards one goal but not the other.

- **Approach planning**: state actions/interventions in simple terms. Use verbs in their base form. For example, *use* (a base form of a verb) *plain, simple, concrete language when speaking with resident*.

- **Re-evaluation**: express results of the re-evaluation of care in simple terms, by saying what happened. Use the present perfect tense for this. For example, *patient has learnt* (present perfect) *to express his basic needs in simple but clear language*. If the re-evaluation shows that you need to set new goals, use the same language and tenses as in goal-setting above. For example, *patient has a knowledge deficit regarding the transmission, complications and treatment of Chlamydia*, or *patient has been diagnosed with breast cancer*.

Activity 7.1

Here is a short summary of the situation of Mrs M. Read it and complete the care plan below. Complete as much as you can and then check with the suggested answer at the end of the book.

Mrs M, 65, has been hospitalized for the second time this month. Her medical record number is ICD-9-CM 348.1 and she is in room 231. She presents a severe loss of self-image and self-esteem due to effects of chemotherapy.

Patient's name

Medical record number

Room number

Date

Problem	Description	Goal

Approach	Assessment	Review (re-evaluation)

Answers See suggested answers on page 198.

How to write portfolios

This section of the chapter examines portfolios as a tool for academic and professional development.

A student portfolio may be defined as a tool to:

- assess a student's performance in a comprehensive manner;
- study the work done by a student;
- identify strengths and weaknesses in the learning path taken by a student;

- analyse recent achievements;
- decide on a course of action to ensure development.

A professional portfolio is also a very important tool in the nursing and midwifery professions. A professional portfolio is a collection of documents that give evidence of a person's professional career, and that can be used as the basis for a person's

- curriculum vitae;
- career path;
- promotion;
- continuous professional development.

Portfolios contain a collection of a student's or a professional's work over a period of time, that are used as evidence of academic or professional development, achievement and needs. The contents of a portfolio will obviously vary depending on whether it is a student or a professional portfolio. The student portfolio will normally contain:

- **a statement of purpose**: the main reasons why you are writing this portfolio;
- **personal information**: name, contact details, other relevant ID;
- **clinical experience**: clinical placements, work experience (including assignments you have written on this);
- **assignments**: a selection of assignments that show the academic progress you have made so far;
- **reflective documents**: a reflective essay (see Chapter 4) critically showing how you have developed since you started your course or your university programme, and your personal development planning – where you have been, where you are, where you would like to be, and how you will get there (skills and knowledge needed);
- **personal development plans** and **action plans**.

The professional portfolio will contain:

- **a statement of purpose**: the main reasons why you are writing this portfolio;
- **personal information**: name, contact details, registration details, other relevant ID;
- **education**: schools, colleges and universities you have previously attended, courses you have taken, other relevant information

> (including copies of certificates, examination results, transcripts, etc.), other professional qualifications;
- record of employment: professional posts within the discipline, professional posts outside the discipline (including copies of job descriptions or brief description of duties and responsibilities);
- professional development: clinical supervision, research and project work, conferences and seminars participated in and attended, memberships of professional bodies (including details), personal development plans;
- reflective documents: a reflective piece of writing critically showing how you have developed since you started your career, and your personal development planning – where you have been, where you are, where you would like to be, and how you will get there (skills and knowledge needed), and action plans.

As you can see, reflective writing is the central document in both kinds of portfolios. In this piece of writing the writer can use their **critical skills** to reflect upon their strengths and weaknesses, to plan their personal growth and to decide on a course of action to pursue their professional development.

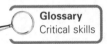
Glossary
Critical skills

A portfolio can be either paper-based or electronic. Both have advantages and disadvantages. Paper-based portfolios are easy to handle and display, and are self-contained products. However, they are also less flexible, less appropriate for documents of various sizes, and more difficult to expand over a long period of time. Electronic portfolios are very flexible and easy to expand, can incorporate documents of almost any size and in any format (e.g. video clips, audio files), but they are dependent on a computer for display. This means that arrangements have to be made in advance to view the portfolio.

Paper-based portfolios can be stored and presented in:

- ring-binders or folders;
- plastic ringers;
- plastic folders;
- tab dividers.

Electronic portfolios can be stored and presented in:

- floppy disks;
- CDs;
- DVDs.

Finally, let us have a look at some of the criteria commonly used to assess a student portfolio. Portfolios are normally assessed in three areas:

- **Organization**: Has the content been logically organized? Do the documents in each section reflect the aims and objectives of the section?
- **Content**: Have the documents been appropriately chosen? Do the documents represent strong evidence of the portfolio owner's knowledge and skills? Does the quality of the document contents evidence their skills and values?
- **Presentation**: Are the entries well-written? Do they evidence problems with spelling and grammar? Does the portfolio look professional? Does it create a positive imagine of the owner?

How to write reports

You will be also asked to write reports as a student and later on as a professional. Simply defined, reports are documents that:

- have a very clear objective and a specific purpose;
- are written for a specific audience;
- have a distinctive structure and layout;
- contain information as well as recommendations.

As you can see, reports are distinctive documents and as such they differ from other genres discussed earlier. A report does not discuss opinions or theories, but presents and analyses information, and makes recommendations upon which the reader is expected to act.

There are different types of reports, and they can be put on a cline ranging from the *academic report* at one end to the *professional report* at the other (Figure 7.2).

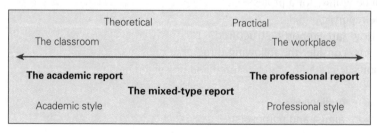

Theoretical   Practical

The classroom   The workplace

←——→

The academic report   **The professional report**

The mixed-type report

Academic style   Professional style

Figure 7.2   The report cline

Now, reports are written for different purposes and with different audiences in mind, both the purpose and audience will determine its content as well as its structure. Lecturers, for example, ask students to write reports as assignments; these will be *academic reports*. As shown in Figure 7.2, the academic report is more theoretical in nature and will observe all the academic conventions that you have analysed in the previous chapters of this book. The report that students may be asked to write after a work placement is an example of an academic report. It is a formal piece of writing, focusing on the theoretical aspects of an issue and its recommendations will result from an analysis of the literature used in preparation for the report. You will be most probably asked to use your placement experience to illustrate the theoretical points you are reporting, but the focus will still be on theory.

The *professional report*, on the other hand, tends to be more practical in nature and aims at solving a given problem or situation. Its recommendations or evaluations will then be orientated to solving the problem or improving the situation analysed. Professional reports normally follow the style of the workplace for which they have been written. In the healthcare sector there are many types of reports produced for and by the National Health Service (NHS) in the UK. There are, for instance, investigation reports that examine the causes of serious problems in the provision of good quality care to patients in the NHS. The main aim here is to make recommendations to solve the problems under investigation. Another example of professional reports is the staff survey report that gathers information to help improve the working lives of care providers within the organization.

Mixed-type reports result from situations where there is a combination of writers, purposes or audiences. For example, a business person who normally writes professional reports may be asked to write a report as an example to be used in a business class. In this case, the purpose of the report – a pedagogical purpose – will require the writer to produce a mixed type report. Similarly, a university student on a work placement, who normally writes academic reports, may be asked to produce a report for the company where he/she is on placement. In this case the writer is a student but he/she will be writing for a professional audience. This again will produce a mixed-type report.

How are reports structured? Before we discuss the structure of reports, consider the following three principles that will give shape to your reports:

- audience;
- aim(s) and purpose(s);
- contents.

So the questions you need to ask at the planning stage are:

- **Who** am I writing this for? What do they know about this? What do they want to do with this report?
- **Why** am I writing this?
- **What** will they need to know to make informed decisions?

These three elements are closely interrelated, and each will influence the others. Thus, if your report is:

- expected to **encourage further thinking** about the issue(s) it examines, then its **findings section** is the most **crucial**;
- an account of something you have **observed**, then its **recommendations section** is the most **vital**;
- on an in-progress **project**, then the sections where it deals with the **evidence** and makes its **recommendations** are **critical**.

Once you have answered these questions and considered how they are related, it is time for you to decide on the different parts of a report. This section will focus on *academic reports* as they will be the most frequently required in your academic life. Your academic reports should have three main sections, the **preliminaries**, the **body** and the **end matter**. The list below shows you the different components of each of these sections, followed by a more detailed discussion of the essential components.

- **Preliminaries**
    - *Cover sheet* (title of report, your name, the name of the institution, the date you produced the report);
    - *Title page* (full title of report, your name);
    - *Acknowledgements* (acknowledge the people who have helped or supported you);
    - *Table of contents* (list different sections together with their page number); and
    - *Abstract/Summary/Executive summary* (an abstract of the complete report: the procedure followed, initial findings, conclusions and recommendations).
- **Body**
    - *Aims and purposes* (why you wrote the report);
    - *Literature review* (critical analysis of the literature related to your report);

- *Methodology* (type of methods used, data collection and ethical issues);
- *Results* (what you found out, using graphs, tables and figures to support text);
- *Analysis* (critical interpretation of results);
- *Conclusions* (the conclusions you arrived at); and
- *Recommendations* (what course of action should be taken considering your conclusions).
- **End matter**
  - *References* (sources cited in your report);
  - *Bibliography* (sources you consulted but did not cite); and
  - *Appendices* (supporting evidence/graphs/statistics etc. that are too long to be included in the body).

Let us consider the most essential components of each of these parts. Obviously, the central element in the preliminaries is the *abstract*, which should summarize:

- The **problem** investigated;
- The **action** taken to investigate the problem;
- The **results** from such an action.

One thing to keep in mind about the abstract is that it is not a kind of introduction, but a summary of the whole report, so don't get tempted to repeat the contents of your introduction here. Your abstract should be concise – in no more than 200 words, and informative at the same time – and it should summarize the points mentioned above.

The components of the body of a report are all important. However, some are more relevant than others depending on what is reported. The methodology and the presentation of the results, for instance, are more relevant to reports on experimental research than those on reviews of the existing literature. While a report can refer to the methodology of a given study or experiment, it may be more difficult to describe and examine the different methods used in different studies in the relevant literature.

This section will analyse those components of the body that are relevant to reports on experiments as well as on a review of the literature. They are:

- Literature review;
- Analysis of results;
- Conclusions; and
- Recommendations.

Activity 7.2

These two texts come from the same report. Compare them and decide which is

1   part of the abstract,
2   part of the introduction of the report.

Text 1

Although simulation as a pedagogical tool has been used in many university programmes, it has been more widely implemented in business and medical degree programmes (Hook, 2003; Morton & Rauen, 2004; Robinson, 2001). In nursing, simulation has been investigated for more than 20 years now, especially in the US academic context. Simulation has been identified as a pedagogical tool that can help nursing students operate in a 'microworld' in which their actions and interactions can be studied, explored, and used for training purposes (Gordon & Cooper, 2004). Patient simulators, for example, give nursing students all the information they need to make clinical decisions.

Text 2

The pedagogical value of simulation in university programmes has been under investigation for the last 30 years. The Nursing and Midwifery Council (NMC) in the UK has now started a pilot programme to investigate the benefits of using simulation to help nursing students to be fit for practice before registration. This report presents the results of researching the previous applications of simulation in various other university degree programmes, examining the results from such applications, and analysing the pedagogical and professional implications of applying simulation in degree programmes. Based on these considerations, the report makes recommendations as to what approaches to implementing simulation in nursing should be followed.

Answers See suggested answers on page 198.

The key section in the body is the literature review. The rest of the sections will be based on the issues discussed in this component. As stated above, the literature review presents a critical analysis (not a summary!) of major works in the field or topic of the report (see also the final section of this chapter below).

The analysis of the results is also another important part of the body of a report. Here you will have to examine the importance and relevance of the results presented in the studies you reviewed in the literature, and also to refer to the implications of the results for the issues about which you are writing.

The next section presents what you can conclude based on the evidence presented in the literature review and the analysis of results. It is important

here to follow the logical principles examined in relation to writing an argument in Chapter 6. A conclusion is only relevant to a discussion as long as it
results from the evidence presented and analysed in that discussion. This is
especially important when you have to make recommendations as they will
be based on your conclusions.

Thus recommendations should establish a logical link between the different issues discussed in the body of the report and the conclusions you
arrived at after analysing the results. The same principles about making
sensible recommendations you examined in relation to the care critique in
Chapter 5 apply here. Figure 7.3 reproduces the relationship between issues,
conclusion and recommendations.

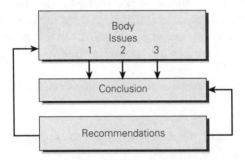

Figure 7.3 The relationship between conclusion and recommendations

In the 'end matter', the last section of a report, the main component is the
list of references. As you may remember from Chapter 1, the list of references
of a report should contain only those sources mentioned in the body of the
report (see also Chapter 10). The bibliography is also important in a report as
it may be used to direct the reader to sources of information you consulted for
the preparation of the report. Although these sources have not been cited in
the body of the report, they can serve as further references to the reader.

Finally, here are some notes on the style of reports. Remember to observe
conventions for referencing and for presenting your final product and if
necessary refer to Chapters 1 (conventions) and 10 (referencing).

- Unlike essays, reports don't always use continuous prose. What is
  more, most reports will combine some prose in the form of short
  paragraphs with bullet points, something which is avoided in essay
  writing.
- Most reports will have numbered headings and sub-headings to
  guide the reader through its contents and to make it easier for
  them to find specific information more quickly and effectively.

Reports will also contain a considerable number of tables, charts and graphs. Before writing, it would be very useful for you to visit the websites of some multinational corporations and download their annual reports to see some good examples. You can access company reports by clicking on 'about us/name of company' or 'company', and then on 'corporate information', or 'investors'. Alternatively, you can consult some of the resources for using tables, charts and graphs listed at the end of this book.

● **How to write research proposals**

Research proposals are another important kind of document you will have to write, especially when you are nearing the end of your course of study or when you start your professional career. You can follow the same organization and structure of research proposals to write your undergraduate dissertation proposal.

Research proposals can serve many different functions; they can help you:

- think through the research project you are planning and envisage possible difficulties;
- get organized;
- think about ways in which difficulties can be overcome;
- anticipate possible results;
- keep you on track once you have started your project.

Research proposals will also help you discuss your ideas with other people; they are a good starting point for discussing your work with other students, your personal tutor and your supervisor. It is important that you keep your proposal as flexible as possible so that you will be able to make room for suggestions you think are worth accepting.

What sections should a research proposal have? This will depend on what type of research you are planning to do. An experimental project will certainly have more sections than a study based on a literature search.

Research has traditionally been divided into:

- **field research**, also called experimental or primary research;
- **desk research**, also called bibliographic or secondary research.

Field research is conducted when you want to obtain new data to answer a specific set of questions about a topic or issue of interest. Questionnaires, interviews, tasks or tests are normally used as data collection instruments. Statistical tests are then used to measure how representative of the population at large your data are. For example, as part of your field research you may want to examine the nursing needs of minority ethnic groups in a given region of your country. You would need to design a questionnaire to use with your chosen sample of that population. You would then need to examine the results from your questionnaires using statistical tests to measure the strength of your results. In the health sciences this type of research, known as **applied research**, often seeks to improve the healthcare of a particular group or the treatment of a particular disease.

A piece of desk research is conducted when you need to analyse data that have already been collected by others. This involves the critical examination of sources of information such as journal articles, books, library databases, reports, and government statistics. You may examine what has been published in connection with your topic so as to be able to evaluate the strength and the weaknesses of our knowledge in that area and suggest gaps in the literature that should be bridged. This is also known as **basic research** in health sciences.

Table 7.3 illustrates the different parts of a research proposal, together with a short description of what should be included in each section. It also indicates whether the section should be part of your proposal, depending on the type of research project you are planning.

How to prepare to write your undergraduate dissertation

This section of the chapter discusses how to *get prepared* to write your undergraduate dissertation. It *does not deal with dissertations* as such, for which you will have to consult your personal tutor or supervisor and other books that specifically deal with dissertation writing. Rather, this section deals with planning and organizing to write the different sections of your dissertation draft.

In your view/experience what parts should an undergraduate dissertation have? (Add more balloons if necessary)

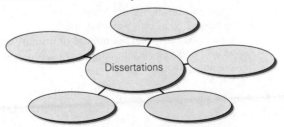

Dissertations

Section	Short description	Type Field	Desk
Title page	Should contain name of university, school/department, your name, student number, the working title of project, your supervisor's name, and the date you are handing it in.	✔	✔
Abstract	Should be a concise summary of your whole proposal. Abstracts are short and should not be confused with introductions.	✔	✔
Introduction	Should provide readers with a description of the background to your research, present its rationale, state the problem you want to examine, specify the steps you will take to do it (objectives) and outline what you will discuss in it (scope).	✔	✔
Literature review	Should briefly explain what we already know about your topic, the main related concepts and theories, whether there are inconsistencies, what needs to be done (gap), and what contribution(s) you expect to make with your research.	✔	✔
Methodology	Should define the type of study you are proposing, access and ethical issues, participants, data collection instruments, and methods of analysis (e.g. statistical tests).	✔	Only briefly explained
Anticipated problems	Should mention problems you may anticipate and consider possible strategies to solve them.	✔	✘
Timeline	Should mention how long you expect the project to last.	✔	✘
Bibliography	Should contain the list of references you have cited in your proposal, the sources you have read but not cited, and also those you intend to read but have not yet had time.	✔	✔

Table 7.3 Sections of a research proposal

Compare your answers with the list shown in Table 7.4. Tick those you included in the spidergram and cross those you did not. You can use this as a checklist for your own work, paying closer attention to those sections for which you have selected a cross.

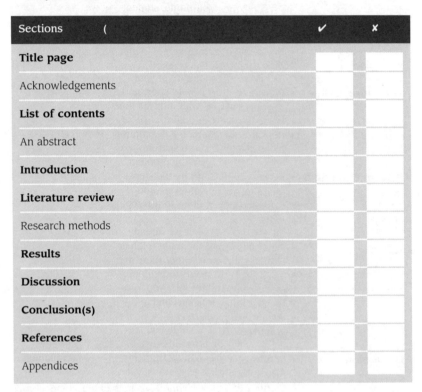

Sections (	✔	✘
Title page		
Acknowledgements		
List of contents		
An abstract		
Introduction		
Literature review		
Research methods		
Results		
Discussion		
Conclusion(s)		
References		
Appendices		

Table 7.4   Sections of a dissertation

Sections in bold are common to both desk-research and field research dissertations. For example, the research methods and results sections will be part of a field research dissertation, but will not normally be part of a desk research one.

The functions of each main section of a dissertation are illustrated in Table 7.5.

There are questions that can help you make sure you have included all the relevant information in each of these sections. Such questions (Table 7.6) can serve two purposes: they can help you plan and get organized before you start writing your dissertation; they can also be used as a checklist after

Section	Main functions
Introduction	• Provides *background* to contextualize the problem your dissertation will focus on; • Presents the *rationale* for your research; • Indicates what *gap* in our knowledge or understanding your dissertation will fill; • States the *objectives* and research questions of your dissertation and its scope.
Literature review	• Presents a *critical analysis* of the work already existing in your research area; • Points to the *gaps* your dissertation will fill; • Indicates the *contributions* your dissertation will make to the field.
Research methods	• Makes reference to the *type of study* (qualitative, quantitative, mixed methods, etc.); • Explain *access* and *confidentiality* issues; • Indicates *arrangements of groups* (control, experimental, etc.); • Describes *instruments for data collection* used; • Explains the *statistical tests* used if applicable.
Results	• Discusses *findings* relating to research questions; • Points to the *salient aspects* of the findings; • Uses *varied methods of presentation* of findings (tables, graphs, etc.).
Discussion	• Confirms or disconfirms your *hypothesis* (field research only); • Clarifies the *research questions* in the light of the results presented; • Discusses the *contribution* of your research.
Conclusion(s)	• Summarizes *discussion* of results; • Clarifies the *implications* of your findings; • Analyses *limitations* of your research; • Suggests areas of *further research*.

Table 7.5   The functions of the main sections of a dissertation

you have produced your first draft. Readers of your dissertation should be able to answer these questions after they have read each part in your dissertation:

Section	Main functions
Introduction	• Where is this problem contextualized? And where can this problem be observed? • Why is this research important? • What is the gap in our knowledge this research will fill? • What steps will be taken to improve the situation? • What aspects of the problem will the research discuss?
Literature review	• What is already known about the field of study? • What are the main concepts in the field? • How are these concepts related? • What theories are the most prominent in the field? • What shortcomings/inconsistencies are there in the field? • What needs to be done? • Why investigate the research problem posed in the study? • What contribution will the study make to the field?
Research methods	• What type of study is this? • Have issues of access to the data and confidentiality been addressed? • What arrangements have been made to the groups studied or the data collected? • What instruments for data collection have been used? • How have the data been analysed?
Results	• How do the findings relate to the research questions? • What are the most salient aspects of the findings?
Discussion	• Does the discussion section illuminate the research questions? • If the research is hypotheses driven, have they been confirmed or rejected? • Does the discussion section analyse the contribution the present research makes?
Conclusion(s)	• Does the conclusion relate the findings and the discussion to the research questions? • Does it examine the implications of the findings? • Does it analyse the limitations of the study? • Does it point to areas of further research?

Table 7.6 A checklist for the main sections of a dissertation

Finally, when you are writing your introduction remember that a good introduction should:

- Be **well-organized** (follow the sequence given in Table 7.4);
- Include **enough detail** to whet the reader's appetite, but should not be too long;
- Specify the **problem** to be researched **clearly**.

When preparing to write the literature review, you will have to read widely to be able to write a good review, and you may find it difficult to organize your notes after so much reading. Here are some organizing and writing tips for you to consider when reading for and writing your review:

- When you read, **keep an annotated bibliography**. An annotated bibliography includes a brief critical synopsis of the contents and contributions made by each of the sources you read.
- **Organize** the **synopses** from the annotated bibliography by theme. Relate synopses that deal with the same or a similar topic or issue together.
- Start **focused reading**. Based on the themes you established, read sources that are directly related to the themes. Avoid reading interesting but unconnected sources.
- **Write individual sections**. Write sections, essays if you prefer, on each of the themes you have identified.
- **Integrate individual sections**. Analyse how the individual sections you have written relate to one another and integrate them, producing longer sections.

Revising the objectives of this chapter

Tick those objectives you feel you have achieved and review those you have not yet managed to accomplish. Then complete the **Achievement Chart** at the back of the book.

In this chapter, you have learnt to

☐ write actions plans

☐ write care plans

☐ prepare, write and choose an appropriate format for portfolios

☐ produce reports

☐ identify effective ways of producing research proposals

☐ plan to start writing your dissertation

Part Three

Working with Texts

In this last part we will work on variation in writing, plagiarism and referencing. First we look at how to provide variety to sentences and to the structure of essays. Then we examine plagiarism and how to avoid it, and finally study the most commonly used systems of referencing in your own discipline.

• Chapter 8: Variety in writing

Chapter 8 works at a micro level of writing. It focuses on how to add variety to sentences, how to use different cohesive devices to improve the flow of the texts, and how to achieve variety in structure within and between paragraphs. It also examines academic writing style.

• Chapter 9: Avoiding plagiarism

In this chapter we deal with a fundamental aspect of writing in an academic environment: plagiarism. The chapter starts by exploring what plagiarism means and why you should avoid it. The chapter then focuses on different strategies to avoid plagiarizing other people's work.

• Chapter 10: Referencing systems

This last chapter explores the reasons for as well as the mechanics of referencing in academic writing. In this chapter, we examine in-text referencing, quotations and reference lists, and then look at how to follow referencing systems in nursing and midwifery. The chapter closes with an examination of the most commonly available bibliographic software, EndNote and RefWorks.

8 Variety in Writing

At the end of this chapter, you should be able to:

▶ recognize different ways of adding variety to your texts
▶ identify different sentence openers
▶ use cohesive devices to support textual variety
▶ recognize structural elements used for adding variety between parts of a text

● Text variety

In this section of the chapter we explore variety in texts. Variety is an important concept in writing as it helps us produce texts that are more interesting and easier to read.

Why does variety matter? Textual variety matters for a number of reasons:

- avoids boredom and encourages readers to keep on reading;
- makes your ideas clearer and sound more interesting;
- shows the relationship between ideas (e.g. main and secondary);
- avoids creating the wrong effect in the reader (e.g. a succession of very short sentences may create suspense).

Text variety can be achieved in a number of ways, and it usually results from a combination of factors. For example, it can be achieved by:

- using **different subject forms**: this will help you avoid overusing the typical 'subject + verb' sentence opener;
- changing the **word order** of some of the sentences: can help you make some ideas more prominent;
- adding **connectives** (e.g. 'and', 'however', etc.): connectives will help you vary your sentence structure and length;
- using **different sentence lengths**: combining different lengths of sentences will help you write texts that are more interesting and attractive to read;
- using **related vocabulary items**: using 'word families' (e.g. to ease, easy, easily) and synonymous expressions (e.g. to ease the pain, to relieve the pain) will help you create a lexical thread in your texts. Related words will also enhance cohesion in your texts (See Chapter 1).

Table 8.1 presents a list of these elements and how they contribute to textual variety. The list can assist you when editing your own texts. These elements will be explored in more detail in the following sections of the chapter.

Text element	Can help you
Subject forms	avoid repetition of sentence openers.
Word order	change emphasis.
Connectives	highlight the relationship between ideas.
Sentence length	make your texts flow more smoothly.
Related vocabulary items	add unity to your texts.

Table 8.1   Elements in text variety

Sentence variety

Varying the structure of the sentences in your texts is also important to attract your reader's attention and encourage them to keep on reading.

One common problem of unattractive texts is that they use the same sentence opener or sentence structure time and time again. For example, if a text only shows the typical sentence opener *subject + verb*, it will produce a monotonous effect and its readers will tire easily. Similarly, if the text is a group of only short and simple sentences, it will read as choppy (broken up) and will lose the interest of its readers.

Table 8.2 shows some of the most common problems connected with sentence variety and offers some alternatives to improve them. The grammar of the sentences is further explained in the section on writing style later in the chapter.

Of the problems listed in Table 8.2, lack of variety of sentence opener, is the most notorious. To avoid repeating the common sentence opener 'subject + verb' vary the form of the subject of your sentences. Here are some of the most common forms that sentences can take as subject:

- Clause: *Although his case was not urgent*, the patient was examined immediately.
- Adverb: *Quickly* and *effectively*, all casualties were treated by the new team of surgeons.

Activity 8.1

Read the following two texts and then answer the questions below:

1 How do you think the texts compare?
2 Which shows more variety?
3 How do you think variety has been achieved in it?
4 Can you underline the elements that have been used to support variety in the text?

Text 1

Nurses can work in many healthcare settings. They can gain experience in all aspects of caring for clients and their families. They can build their professional career in many different ways. They may choose to become clinical specialists or consultant nurses, or they can opt for managerial positions as a head of nursing services or supervisor of other nurses. They may even prefer to pursue an academic career in education and research. These are just a few examples of the opportunities that nurses currently have to develop their professional interests.

Text 2

Nurses can work in many healthcare settings, which gives them the opportunity to gain experience in all aspects of caring for clients and their families. Nurses can thus build their professional career in many different ways. For instance, they may choose to become clinical specialists or consultant nurses, or they can opt for managerial positions as a head of nursing services or supervisor of other nurses. For the more academic oriented ones, there are also opportunities in education and research. These are just a few examples of the opportunities that nurses currently have to develop their professional interests.

Answers See suggested answers on page 198.

- Infinitive phrase: *To gain a deeper understanding of the issue*, the midwife gathered as much information as she possibly could.
- Participial phrase: *Hoping to gain a deeper understanding of the issue*, the midwife gathered as much information as she possibly could.
- Nominalization: *A decision about the case* was not made until the small hours of the following day.
- Cleft-sentences: *It was his weight loss* that called everyone's attention.

Problem	Alternative 1	Alternative 2
Choppy sentences	Use **co-ordination** (if ideas are of equal value): 'and', 'but', 'or', 'so', etc.	Use **subordination** (if one idea is dependent on the other): 'when', 'while', 'because', etc.
Same subject in various consecutive sentences	**Replace** the subject for a pronoun.	Use **relative pronouns**: 'who', 'which', 'that'.
Subject + verb pattern in various consecutive sentences	Use a **preposition** to start the sentence: **After** completing the form, the patient was directed to ...	Use a **participle** to start the sentence: **Having completed** the form, the patient was directed to ...

Table 8.2 Problems with sentence structure

Activity 8.2

Read the following text and underline the forms of the subject that have been used to add variety to the text.

Cutting and repairing an episiotomy, and repairing vaginal/perineal lacerations were each proposed and retained as basic skills. Repairing a cervical laceration was proposed and retained as an additional skill. There is considerable Grade I evidence that avoiding episiotomy enhances both short- and long-term perineal integrity, supporting the midwifery philosophy of non-intervention. This evidence is counter-balanced by other Grade I evidence that restricting the use of episiotomy increases the risk of anterior perineal trauma.

Answers See suggested answers on page 199.

● Word order

Changing the word order of a sentence will also add variety to your text. It will also help you change the emphasis of a sentence, while calling the reader's attention to the point being made in that part.

Consider the following two examples:

1 She never thought she would be promoted so quickly.
2 Never did she think she would be promoted so quickly.

In (1) the focus of information attention is placed on the second part of the sentence (quick promotion). In sentence (2), on the other hand, the emphasis falls on how unexpected the promotion was for her.

Consider these other two examples:

3 The doctor saw her patients in ward 2 yesterday morning.
4 Yesterday morning the doctor saw her patients in ward 2.

While the focus of attention is on what happened in sentence (3), in sentence (4) it is on when it happened.

It is important to remember though that when you change the word order of your sentences, you also change their focus of attention. Make sure there is a good reason for doing this, and that the point you are trying to make by changing the focus of attention is clear and justifiable. Otherwise, you may create confusion in your readers.

● Cohesive variety

Cohesion is what holds a text together (see Chapters 2 and 5). Cohesion is necessary not only between sentences, but also between paragraphs. Cohesive variety can be achieved by using:

- words that are related (e.g. synonymous expressions);
- cohesive devices (e.g. finally);
- related concepts;
- reference to previously mentioned points (e.g. this, that);
- substitution (e.g. substituting 'nurses' by the personal pronoun 'they').

Table 8.3 shows examples of how these elements can be used to achieve cohesiveness. Use the list to help you edit your own texts.

● Structural variety in paragraphs

The term structural variety encompasses all the other aspects of variety that you have examined in the previous sections. This section shows you how

Cohesive element	Example
Related words	Surgical treatment for gynaecological cancer raises particular difficulties in relation to *altered fertility*, *changes in body image* and *sexual dysfunction*. These *problems* may, in turn, trigger a significant life crisis for the entire family. (Maughan, Heyman & Matthews, 2002: 27)
Cohesive devices	*Although* sleep disturbance is the most important and bothersome symptom experienced by these patients, there are few documented interventional studies that have addressed this problem. *Thus*, there is a need to develop effective methods to manage sleep disturbance of ESRD patients. (Tsaya & Chen, 2003: 1)
Related concepts	All human beings need stimulation to keep their *brain functioning* in a normal way. Deprivation of stimulation leads to a *deterioration of behaviour*. There is a considerable risk that the patient in the final stage of *dementia* will get too little stimulation. (Norberg, Melin & Asplund, 2003: 473)
This, **that**, **these**, **those** (to refer to previously mentioned points/ ideas)	Surgical treatment for gynaecological cancer raises particular difficulties in relation to altered fertility, changes in body image and sexual dysfunction. *These* problems may, in turn, trigger a significant life crisis for the entire family. (Maughan, Heyman, & Matthews, 2002: 27)
Substitution	Managers of the units were asked to inform *staff and nurses* during the ward meeting about the purpose of the investigation and asked *them* to take part in it. The questionnaires were distributed in a sealed envelop including an introductory letter and *they* were told that *their* anonymity would be preserved. (Tummers, van Merode & Landeweerd, 2003: 845)

Table 8.3 Cohesive elements in texts

Activity 8.3

Read the following text and underline the elements that have been used to achieve cohesiveness:

As pressure to control hospital costs has intensified, the need to deliver the best nursing care in the most economical way has grown. Internationally research reviews show the benefits of home care. For example, dialysis patients can be reunited with their families and hospital beds used only when really necessary. In addition, by reducing hospital stays, governments undoubtedly save thousands of dollars. Nevertheless, it is not possible for professionals and policy-makers to estimate the resource implications of in-home services in Hong Kong unless systematic research is undertaken. (Luk, 2002: 269)

Answers See suggested answers on page 199.

they all work together to keep the structure within and between paragraphs attractive to your readers and we should examine how to:

- combine long and short sentences within paragraphs;
- provide logical connections between paragraphs.

It is important to **combine short and long sentences** in the same paragraph. Too many long sentences would make reading the text more demanding and may lead to confusion. Too many short sentences, on the other hand, may create a choppy effect in your text. A long sentence should be followed by a short one, especially if another long sentence will follow afterwards.

The short sentence may have several functions. It may:

- summarize the ideas in the previous sentence;
- provide a link between two long sentences;
- mark a transition between the topics of two long sentences.

Providing **logical connections or relationships between paragraphs** is

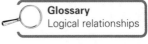
Glossary
Logical relationships

another way of adding textual variety, while also making transitions between the parts of your text smoother. Logical connections can be marked by a word (similarly), a phrase (on the other hand) or a whole sentence.

You should provide logical connections between paragraphs when you want to:

Activity 8.4

Read the following texts and choose one of the labels below to define the function of the sentence in italics in each of them. There is one too many labels.

Summarize	Link	Mark a transition

Text 1

Several studies suggest that brief interventions do not significantly contribute to smoking cessation during pregnancy and have concluded that interventions may benefit the fetus but their medium term effects on helping mothers stop smoking are inconclusive. *This seems to indicate that to be effective smoking cessation intervention should consider both the fetus and the mother.* It seems reasonable to suggest that programmes of sustained support would need to be implemented so as to help smokers not only during pregnancy but also after giving birth.

Text 2

Client-centred care, which sees the client as a holistic individual, is one of the basic principles that a nurse should learn as it underlies both the theory and the practice of nursing care. *To provide client-centred care, nurses should recognize culture-sensitive practices and their relation to social cultures.* Societal characteristics are important sources of information for nurses to be able to make informed decisions in their daily practice as these should result from their reflection on practice and respect for ethnicity, culture and differences.

Answers See suggested answers on page 199.

- show comparison or contrast between the two parts of your text (e.g. using 'however' for contrast and 'similarly' for comparison);
- enumerate reasons or examples;
- produce a counterargument (e.g. using a concession: although these cases have clearly been reviewed, there are still some inconclusive results that require further examination).

Writing style

All the different elements we discussed in the previous sections constitute what we call 'writing style'. They can be grouped into three basic principles that should guide your academic writing:

Activity 8.5

Read the following texts and underline the logical connections used. In some cases, you don't have the preceding text but you should still be able to identify the logical connection.

Text 1
In contrast to this prevailing view of women as objects, many international leaders and agencies have taken action to promote women as persons with full human rights, beginning with the female child. (Thompson, 2002: 189)

Text 2
Psychiatric and Social Work pre-admission assessments have long-standing histories as requirements of UK Mental Health Acts (1983). Pre-admission nursing assessment has no such obvious legal authority; however, the practice is commonplace for most, if not all, Medium and High Security Hospitals.
  Despite the widespread nature of this practice, preadmission nursing assessments have received little descriptive or research attention in forensic mental health. (Watt *et al.*, 2003: 645)

Text 3
The women in the midwifery group were seen by an obstetrician during their initial visit to the midwives' clinic and at 36 weeks gestation to confirm their low-risk status.
  Apart from the two mandatory obstetrician visits, the midwives made autonomous decisions on the care they provided. They made referrals to, or consulted with, obstetricians and other health team members when the need arose. (Harvey *et al.*, 2002: 262)

Answers See suggested answers on page 200.

- Simplicity;
- Brevity;
- Logic.

Each of these principles can be achieved in a number of ways. *Simplicity*, for example, has to do with sentence length and choice of words. *Logic* is the result of careful planning, using the right connectives and following grammatical principles such as agreement. We will now analyse each of these principles in more detail.

Simplicity
One way of keeping your writing simple is by keeping an eye on the length of

your sentences. This of course doesn't mean that all your sentences should be short and simple. As we said above, a succession of short sentences will give your text a choppy style or create an effect of suspense you surely want to avoid in your academic essays. On the other hand, too many complex sentences together will tire your reader. What you should try and do is to combine short and long sentences, which will add variety to your text, making it easy and pleasant to read. Compare these three examples:

Example 1: A succession of short sentences

Many studies have produced inconclusive evidence in relation to smoking cessation during pregnancy (e.g. Kelley *et al.*, 2001; Melvin *et al.*, 2000; Melvin & Gaffney, 2004). Several of these studies suggest that brief interventions do not contribute to smoking cessation during pregnancy (Fiore *et al.*, 2000; Lumley *et al.*, 2004). Lawrence *et al.* (2005) have forcefully concluded that some programmes may benefit the foetus but not the mother. This seems to indicate that smoking cessation in pregnancy is unsuccessful because support to the woman is only occasional and lacks structure. Programmes of sustained support would need to be implemented during pregnancy and after birth. These programmes should then be structured in a way that offers both in-pregnancy and postpartum support.

Example 2: A succession of long and complex sentences

Although many studies have produced inconclusive evidence in relation to smoking cessation during pregnancy (e.g. Kelley *et al.*, 2001; Melvin *et al.*, 2000; Melvin & Gaffney, 2004), several seem to suggest that brief interventions do not contribute to smoking cessation during pregnancy (Fiore *et al.*, 2000; Lumley *et al.*, 2004). Lawrence *et al.* (2005) have forcefully concluded that some programmes may benefit the foetus but not the mother, which seems to indicate that smoking cessation in pregnancy is unsuccessful because support to the woman is only occasional and lacks structure and thus programmes of sustained support would need to be implemented during pregnancy and after birth, and should be structured in a way that offers both in-pregnancy and postpartum support.

Example 3: A combination of short and long sentences

Many studies have produced inconclusive evidence in relation to smoking cessation during pregnancy (e.g. Kelley *et al.*, 2001; Melvin *et al.*, 2000; Melvin & Gaffney, 2004). Several of these studies suggest that brief interventions do not contribute to smoking cessation during pregnancy (Fiore *et al.*, 2000; Lumley *et al.*, 2004). Lawrence *et al.* (2005) have forcefully concluded that some programmes may benefit the foetus but not the mother, which seems to indicate that smoking cessation in pregnancy is unsuccessful because support to the woman is only occasional and lacks structure. Thus, programmes of sustained support would need to be implemented during pregnancy as well as after birth. These programmes should then be structured in a way that offers both in-pregnancy and postpartum support.

Choice of words will also contribute to keeping your style simple. This doesn't mean that you should avoid using 'technical vocabulary' that is part of the lexis of your discipline. Technical words may first appear complex, but these are the words your readers expect to find in your writing. What is more, technical words are very difficult to be replaced as they have become part of the technical vocabulary used to write about your discipline. As opposed to general and vague words (e.g. thing, it, nice), accurate and specific words will always contribute positively to your writing style. If this is the first time you're writing an assignment on a topic you are not very familiar with, it is always a good idea to start collecting words that recur in your reading sources. These words make up the core technical vocabulary that you will need to use for your writing to be accurate and precise. Look at the following two examples; technical or precise words in the first text have been underlined and replaced by less accurate ones in example 2.

Example 1: Accurate and precise

Post partum haemorrhage (PPH) has been identified as one of the main complications of the third stage which accounts for the highest maternal mortality and morbidity. As demonstrated in this care, there is compelling evidence that lends support to the benefits of active management of the third stage.

Example 2: General and vague

Blood loss after birth has been identified as one the main things that may happen in the third stage which accounts for the highest level of death and disease. As demonstrated in this care, there are a lot of examples that show the benefits of active participation of the midwife in the third stage.

Brevity

This is also connected to simplicity and to a principle of economy that will improve the readability of your writing. Brevity also has to do with the selection and organization principles you studied in Chapter 1. The more focused your writing becomes, that is free from loosely connected ideas and words, the more effective the impact it will create on readers. Keep it simple and avoid superfluous elements that will add words but no meaning to your sentences.

Logic

Logic also depends on selection and organization. A logical writing style is one in which the ideas – and the sentences used to express those ideas – flow smoothly. As we discussed above, if the first idea in your paragraph is complex and has been presented in a complex sentence, you will need to flesh out its meaning in two or probably three short and simple sentences. Coupled with this combination, you will need connectives to reinforce the logical organization of your writing.

Agreement between subject and verb will also make your writing more logical and cohesive. If the subject and the verb of a sentence don't agree, this will then create confusion in the reader's mind. Consider the following example:

> **Poor style**: 'Doctor Jones, after seeing all his patients, go home.'
> (Who goes home? The doctor or his patients?)
> **Improved**: 'Doctor Jones, after seeing all his patients, goes home.'

Similarly, if the subject of a sentence is later referred to by a pronoun that doesn't agree with it, it will also create confusion, making your writing less logical. Consider this other example:

> **Poor style**: 'Nurses will always make sure that his clients receive the most beneficial care.' (Who is he?)
> **Improved**: 'Nurses will always make sure that their clients receive the most beneficial care.'

Finally, the way you structure your sentences will also contribute positively to your style. Avoid:

- starting sentences with a connective, especially with 'and', 'but' or 'because';
- finishing sentences with prepositions; and
- splitting infinitives.

The following examples show you how these problems can be easily avoided to enhance your writing style:

Example 1: Starting sentences with a connective

Poor style: There are a few intervention programmes to treat clients with a dual diagnosis. **But** they are relatively new and have not been objectively evaluated for their effectiveness. **And** increasing attention to these issues is being paid in some countries and, as a result, several integrated approach treatment programmes have been established.

Improved: There are a few intervention programmes to treat clients with a dual diagnosis. However, they are relatively new and have not been objectively evaluated for their effectiveness. In some countries increasing attention to these issues is being paid and, as a result, several integrated approach treatment programmes have been established.

Example 2: Finishing sentences with prepositions

Poor style: These are some of the issues they have been writing **about**.

Improved: These are some of the issues **about which** they have been writing.

Example 3: Splitting infinitives

Poor style: The nurse wanted **to systematically examine** the care that patients received in that ward.

Improved: The nurse wanted **to examine systematically** the care that patients received in that ward.

● Grammar and English use

This last section of the chapter deals with some of the main grammar and language-use problems that many students experience when writing academically. We will look at sentence grammar, and for easy referencing these problems are examined in the form of a trouble-shooting list (Table 8.4). If you feel you need more detail on any of these topics, see the Glossary of Key Terms and the list of Further Readings and Resources at the end of the book.

Sentence grammar	Explanation	Example
Co-ordination	Co-ordination refers to the process of putting two or more ideas of **equal value** together. They could be written as separate sentences and would still make sense. The main co-ordinators are: AND, BUT, SO, OR.	Patients were administered their medication regularly **and** were given the list of activities they had to carry out on a daily basis.
Subordination	Subordination refers to putting two or more unequal ideas **(one is dependent, D, on the other)** together. If written separately, one would not make complete sense. Some subordinators include: although, unless, if, because, etc.	**Because** she was so tired at the end of the shift (D), she decided to go straight into bed.
Clause	A group of words, one of which is a finite (conjugated) verb.	**At the end of the shift she was so tired that** (1) **she decided to go straight into bed** (2).
Phrase	A group of words without a finite verb	**A group of student midwives**
Infinitive phrase	A phrase whose main word is an infinitive verb.	**To support his patient emotionally** was all that the GP worried about at that moment.

Sentence grammar	Explanation	Example
Participial phrase	A phrase whose main word is an -ed or -ing word, or a word that has the same form as the past participle of irregular verbs (e.g. hidden).	**Hidden under a pile of other forms**, his admission form laid on the desk.
Prepositional phrase	A phrase whose main word is a preposition.	**On performing a pelvic examination**, she discovered the pregnancy was ectopic.
Nominalization	It refers to the process by which a verb or adjective is turned into a noun, resulting in an impersonal structure.	There is **a demand** for further discussions about pregnancy termination.
Cleft-sentences	Sentences that have two parts (and two finite verbs). They are useful to call the reader's attention to the first part of the sentence.	**What we now need** are actions more than words.
Fragment	A phrase or incomplete sentence which is punctuated as a complete sentence would.	**As she was experiencing acute pain and heavy bleeding**.

Table 8.4 Sentence grammar

Revising the objectives of this chapter

Tick those objectives you feel you have achieved and review those you have not yet managed to accomplish. Then complete the **Achievement Chart** at the back of the book.

In this chapter you have learnt to:

☐ recognize different ways of adding variety to your texts

☐ identify different sentence openers

☐ use cohesive devices to support textual variety

☐ recognize structural elements used for adding variety between parts of a text

9 Avoiding Plagiarism

● **Exploring plagiarism**

What do you already know about plagiarism? Complete

Glossary
Plagiarism

the diagram below with some words or phrases you associate with it.

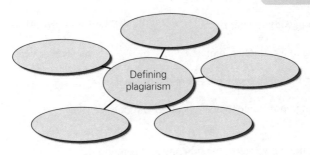

Defining plagiarism

Now read the definitions of plagiarism below. Look especially at the words in bold. Did you write any of these words in your diagram?

According to the *Merriam-Webster Online Dictionary*, to 'plagiarize' means

(1) to **steal** and **pass off** (the ideas or words of another) as one's own
(2 to use (another's production) **without crediting** the source
(3) to commit **literary theft**
(4) to present as new and original an idea or product **derived from** an existing source.

In other words, plagiarism is an **act of fraud**. It involves both **stealing** someone else's work and **lying** about it afterward.

Source: 'What is Plagiarism', Turnitin.com

As the definition says, plagiarism comprises two acts: stealing (somebody else's work) and lying (about it) afterwards. You can avoid plagiarism by being academically honest. Don't steal, and don't lie.

Plagiarism may take many different forms and sometimes students plagiarize without knowing. You could be severely penalized for plagiarism if you do any of the following. Look at the list in Table 9.1 and tick those you can identify as plagiarism and cross those you didn't know about.

Acts	Knew (✔)	Didn't know (✘)
1 Handing in somebody else's work as your own.		
2 Buying or borrowing somebody else's work.		
3 Paying somebody to write for you.		
4 Copying without citing.		
5 Failing to use quotation marks.		
6 Changing only a few words from the original.		
7 Building upon somebody else's ideas without giving credit.		
8 Changing the words in the original but keeping the essential ideas without citing.		
9 Paraphrasing without citing.		

Table 9.1   Acts of plagiarism

Some of these acts can be more easily identified as plagiarism than others. For instance, you may think that *paying somebody to write for you* (item 3) is dishonest but not plagiarism. However, if you do this you are buying somebody else's ideas and words and then pretending they are your own. This *is* plagiarism.

Changing only a few words from the original (item 6) is another form of plagiarism you may not be so sure about. But if you change just a few words without acknowledging the original source, the words are yours but the ideas are certainly not. This is similar to item 8 – *Changing the words in the original but keeping the essential ideas without citing.*

Why do students plagiarize? Some believe that they are incapable of producing work worth reading or worth a good mark. They cannot see themselves prepared to meet their tutors' expectations, so they plagiarise in the hope that they will get a passing mark. Others find it contradictory that, while they have to produce work with a certain degree of originality, they still have to reference previous work in the field (see Chapter 10).

The rest of this chapter deals with strategies for avoiding plagiarism. More specifically, you will look at strategies for dealing with established definitions and concepts, and paraphrasing.

Activity 9.1

You will read one original text and three other texts that have incorporated the original one. Determine which of the three texts plagiarizes and which does not. Be prepared to back up your choices.

Original text
'Despite the difficulties faced by male partners of seriously ill women, their needs may not be recognised. Rees *et al.* (1998) assessed the information needs of nine male partners of women with breast cancer, using focus group methodology. They found that partners varied considerably in their information needs, but that health professionals generally ignored their information needs. Although this study provides a valuable insight into the information needs of partners and health professional responses, the results cannot necessarily be generalised because of the small size of the sample.' (Maughan *et al.*, 2002: 28)

Text 1
Several studies have suggested that the difficulties faced by male partners of seriously ill women may not be recognised (Rees *et al.*, 1998; Maughan *et al.*, 2002).

Text 2
In a small study of the information needs of male partners of seriously ill women, Rees et al. (1998, cited in Maughan *et al.*, 2002: 28) found that health professionals tended to pay little attention to these men's needs.

Text 3
Maughan et al. (2002) state that although male partners of seriously ill women face difficulties, their needs may not be acknowledged.

Answers See suggested answers on page 200.

● Dealing with definitions and concepts

One common misconception about referencing and **paraphrasing** is thinking you cannot 'reproduce' what others have already said because if you do, your work will lack 'originality'. However, sometimes you are better off reproducing what others before you have said. You just have to make sure you do it properly.

One such case is when dealing with established concepts in the field you are researching. If, for example, you are working with the concept of 'reflection' in nursing, people reading your essay would probably expect you to refer to Gibbs' well-established model. Similarly, if your essay was on 'problem-based nursing', you would need to make reference to problem-based learning components and problem-solving processes. These cases allow you to show or display your knowledge of the field and its main contributors (also see Chapter 10).

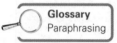

Glossary
Paraphrasing

Another reason for reproducing established ideas and concepts is connected with 'specificity'. Some definitions are highly technical and specific and a paraphrase may not cover all the specific aspects or may fail to convey the same meanings. Think, for example, how difficult it would be to provide synonymous words or phrases for 'fertilisation', 'fertility', 'fertilized' in the following definition:

> In Vitro Fertilisation (IVF) is one of several assisted conception techniques available to help people with fertility problems to have a baby. It involves an egg being surgically removed from the ovary and fertilised outside the body. (*Health Encyclopaedia*, NHS Direct Online)

Providing a new working definition of IVF may prove not only difficult but also unnecessary. Definitions which have been accepted by the professional community have the purpose of making it possible for community members to communicate in an economical and effortless way.

It is important to remember that, to avoid plagiarism, you will need to quote the source from which you took the given definition, as shown above in relation to IVF. For a discussion and explanation of how to quote sources correctly, see Chapter 10.

● Paraphrasing

Paraphrasing is an effective way of using your own words to report what others have said, and offers the possibility of adding variety to your text. A

Activity 9.2

Read the following definition of Chlamydia and decide if the writers of texts 1 and 2 have made the right choice when paraphrasing the definition in their texts. What would you have done?

Definition
'Chlamydia is a common sexually transmitted disease (STD) caused by the bacterium, Chlamydia trachomatis, which can damage a woman's reproductive organs.' (*Health Encyclopaedia*, NHS Direct Online)

Text 1
Chlamydia, an infection that is sexually transmitted, is caused by the bacterium Chlamydia trachomatis.

Text 2
An STD caused by a bacterium, Chlamydia can damage a woman's reproductive organs.

Answers See suggested answers on page 201.

text that is heavily quoted from other sources not only lacks originality but is also uninviting to read. A healthy combination of quotations, in-text referencing (see Chapter 10) and paraphrasing will make a text more attractive to the reader.

But you must keep in mind that changing only a few words from the original does not represent paraphrasing and may be considered plagiarism (see 9.1 the first section of this chapter). When you paraphrase you change the words and sometimes the structure of the original (the form of the quote) but keep the original meanings intact. Paraphrasing thus entails summarizing and referencing. The paraphrase should be shorter and normally more focused than the original text, and for this it is always a good idea to try and concentrate on one central idea to paraphrase. The resulting paraphrase should also acknowledge the source where the original text was found. Here are some ideas to practise paraphrasing original texts:

- Read the original text until you are sure you understand it fully;
- Count the number of words in the original or use the word-count function if you are reading an online document;
- Underline or highlight main and secondary ideas;
- Focus on the main ideas;
- Write the main ideas in your own words;

- Compare your paraphrase with the original;
- If you have used more than 10% of the words in the original, it is NOT a paraphrase and you must go back to reading the original again.

Let us look at the example shown in Table 9.2. In this example first read the original text, then a paraphrase of the original and finally a plagiarized version.

Original	Reported
'Midwifery care is *personalized* care. Within the parameter of safety the midwife upholds, she recognizes wellness as an amorphous state with periodic deviations from normal; her task is to decipher the unique and fluid patterns of each mother's well-being. The more thorough and continuous her care, the more likely she will be to detect a complication at its inception. And the better she and the mother communicate, the more readily will they develop and implement a solution.' (Davis 2004, p. 5) [77 words]	**Paraphrased ✔** One essential responsibility of the midwife is to safely discover patterns of well-being that are individual to each of her clients. This, supported by on-going care and good communication, will allow her to discover complications early and solve them promptly. (Davis 2004, p. 5) [40 words] **Plagiarized ✗** Midwives offer *personalized* care. Midwives' main task is to be able to recognize the patterns of well-being of their clients. To detect complications as soon as they start and to readily implement solutions, midwives should provide continuous care and establish a relationship based on good communication with each of their clients. [51 words]

Table 9.2 Paraphrasing vs plagiarism

Notice that the plagiarized version not only uses many words that are the same as in the original (underlined in the plagiarized version), but also **fails to acknowledge the original source**. It shows the two features of plagiarism discussed earlier in the chapter: it *steals* and it *lies*.

Let us examine another example. The original text below is followed by two other versions, in which the lifted (plagiarized) text in the new versions has been underlined. Comments on the two new versions are given below the texts.

ORIGINAL TEXT

'The midwives in this context appeared to define themselves as advocates for the individual woman, and not as advocates or caregivers for the family as a whole. This can be interpreted as a deviation from an ideology of caring for the family as a whole, implemented in routines of educational programmes for couples antenatally and encouragement of family participation during delivery for Swedish couples. In addition, the midwives often used the word "we" and spoke of themselves as representatives of the Swedish health care system and/or society, versus the word "them" used when speaking about immigrants from traditionally FGM practising cultures, thus illustrating an impression of polarisation.' (Widmark, Tishelman and Ahlberg, 2002: 122)

Version 1	Version 2
The midwives in the Swedish study approached their professional task as providers of care for the individual woman only. This can be analysed as a deviation from the idea that midwives should care for the family as a whole and encourage families to participate in the process of delivery. Besides, the midwives used the pronoun 'we' as representing the Swedish health care system as opposed to the word 'them' when they spoke about immigrants from traditionally female genital mutilation (FGM) practising cultures.	In their study of a group of Swedish midwives, Widmark, Tishelman and Ahlberg (2002: 122) found that the midwives they observed showed a different approach to their professional tasks. This group of midwives preferred a more woman-only oriented approach to providing care, which differed from the traditional family-oriented approach. They also noted that the midwives polarised the descriptions of their relationship with their clients by referring to themselves as representatives of the Swedish health care system with the pronoun 'we', and their FGM practising clients with the pronoun 'them'.
Comments	**Comments**
This is a clear example of a plagiarized text. Except for the first sentence which has been minimally changed, the text consists of almost entirely lifted text. The changes here can be said to be 'cosmetic changes' and there are no bibliographical references to the original text.	This is an example of a good paraphrase. It shows a change not only in the words but also the structures used in the original text. But it has still managed to keep the same meanings as in the original.

You can signpost your paraphrase by using:

- A phrase that refers to the original source (see first sentence of version 2 above);
- An appropriate verb or verb phrase (e.g. suggest, criticize, contradict, etc.) (see the following section).

Activity 9.3

Read the original text and the lifted version. What changes would you make to change the lifted version into a paraphrase?

Original text
'The introduction of a funded midwifery pilot programme in a community where midwifery was not otherwise available provided a unique opportunity to compare the quality of midwifery care with existing maternity services for women at low obstetric risk. The safety of midwifery practice was a major concern in a region that had not experienced midwifery services'. (Harvey *et al.*, 2002: 261)

Lifted version
A funded pilot programme in midwifery support in a community where this support was not available provided the authors an excellent opportunity to compare this service with that of existing maternity services for women at low obstetric risk. One of the major concerns in the region, probably as a result of not having this kind of care before, related to safety.

Answers See suggested answers on page 201.

● Grammar and English use

In Tables 9.3–9.5, you will find more about paraphrasing. Table 9.3 deals with structural paraphrase and Table 9.4 with lexical paraphrase. Table 9.5 explains signposting paraphrase. If you feel you need more detail on any of these topics, see the Glossary of Key Terms and the list of Further Readings and Resources at the end of the book.

Structural paraphrase
It is sometimes difficult to change the structure of the original text without changing its meaning. However, a paraphrase does not follow the original structure, so you must learn ways of changing the structure while keeping the original ideas and concepts. The examples in the following table should give you an idea of how structural paraphrase works.

Change	Details	Example
The order of the parts of the sentence	Adverbials can be moved to front position with only a little change in meaning.	**Original**: They required a rest after their 48-hour shift. **Paraphrase**: After working for 2 days, they needed to rest.
The voice of the original text	From active to passive or from passive to active.	**O**: They provide patient care on an on-going basis. **P**: Continuous care is provided to patients.
The length of the sentences (1)	Join ideas together to make the new sentence shorter and more concise.	**O**: Not only will they work long hours, but they will also earn less. **P**: They will be asked to work longer, but will get less money.
The length of the sentences (2)	Alternatively, you may want to expand phrases for clarity.	**O**: Not having worked in the private sector before, the midwife was unsure of some of the regulations. **P**: The midwife had not worked in the private sector before so she was unclear about some regulations.
The length of the sentences (3)	Abridge a clause to a phrase (but see dangling modifiers in Chapter 1.)	**O**: When they entered the operating theatre, the patient was ready for the operation. **P**: On entering the operating theatre, they found their patient ready for the operation.
Change connectives	Use similar connectives from the same class (AND, SO, BUT, OR).	**O**: The nurse had finished his shift but stayed on to help. **P**: Although he had finished his shift, the nurse stayed on and helped.

Table 9.3 Structural paraphrase

Lexical paraphrase

It may also be difficult to change the words of the original text without changing its meaning. However, as with the structure of a text, you must try and maintain the original meanings. Also remember to leave shared language (language that is not specific to the original text, e.g. 'nurses' or 'midwives') unchanged. Be aware that it may not be possible to change very specific vocabulary items.

Change	Details	Example
Individual words using synonymous expressions	Use a thesaurus and a dictionary.	**Original**: Stopping the habit is essential to the pregnant smoker. **Paraphrase**: It is crucial for the pregnant woman to stop smoking.
Word forms	Nouns to verbs, verbs to nouns, adjectives to adverbs.	**O**: To discover a complication at its inception is fundamental in the health sciences. **P**: The early discovery of complications is an essential aspect of health sciences.

Table 9.4 Lexical paraphrase

Signposting paraphrase

Introduce your paraphrase by using a phrase that links your text to the original or an appropriate verb. Remember to use verbs that show your analytical ability. The table below show you some examples.

Signposting phrase/verb	Example
In (their/his/her) (study/research/work/essay),	**In her 1994 study**, Markus showed that ...
According to....,	**According to Davis's study** (2004), effective communication between the midwife and her client ...
In line with	**In line with** the framework for analysis described by Peterson (2003: 34) as ...
Argue	Peterson (2003: 34) **argues** that a convincing way of ...
Claim	Widmark, Tishelman and Ahlberg (2002) **claim** that their group of midwives polarized ...

Signposting phrase/verb	Example
Observe	Davis (2004) **observes** that early detection of complications will result in ...
Prove	In her study, Campbell (2004) **proved** that most of the methods previously used to determine the degree of ...
Reject	Lawrence *et al.* (2005: 115) seem to **reject** the idea that as administered at present smoking cessation programmes can have any long-term effect on the pregnant smoker.
Suggest	Aston *et al.* (2006) **suggest** that regular interdisciplinary surgical morning meetings (SMM) can contribute to interdisciplinary communication significantly.

Table 9.5   Signposting paraphrase

Revising the objectives of this chapter

Tick those objectives you feel you have achieved and review those you have not yet managed to accomplish. Then, complete the **Achievement Chart** at the back of the book.

In this chapter, you have learnt to:

☐ recognize what constitutes plagiarism and what does not

☐ deal with definitions and concepts already well-established in your field

☐ paraphrase other people's ideas and words without plagia-rising

10 Referencing Systems

At the end of this chapter, you should be able to:

▶ recognize the basic principles of referencing
▶ identify the main referencing conventions of the Harvard, the APA and the Vancouver systems
▶ recognize the basic uses of bibliographic software programmes

● The basics of referencing

Referencing is an essential part of academic writing. Many of your ideas and arguments will need to be

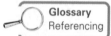
Glossary
Referencing

supported by the ideas or arguments presented by others before you. References provide

---

Activity 10.1

Use the following labels to identify the purpose(s) of referencing in the texts below. One text may accommodate more than one label.

1 **Anchoring the text in the field**
2 **Supporting ideas**
3 **Adding credibility**
4 **Building an argument**

Text A
  Reflection has been identified as an extremely useful skill for nurses (Durgahee, 1996; Johns, 1996; Mountford & Rogers, 1996). Schon (1991), for example, defines reflection as learning from events experienced during a practical professional experience.

Text B
  Reflection is considered an appropriate vehicle for the analysis of professional practice. This analysis helps professionals understand the nature of their work and adopt a critical approach to their professional activity (Gould & Masters, 2004).

Text C
  Many arguments have been advanced in favour of the benefits of returning a patient with a stroke to the open plan unit (Brown, 1999; Thompson, 2004; Willis, 2002). These include the positive support reported by the patients and the quality of the follow-up care. However, the advantages of allowing patients with a stroke to stay in the same room have not been fully examined (Allen, 2001).

Answers See suggested answers on page 201.

a link between your work and the work others have previously done, showing your readers that your ideas are well-founded. Used in this way, references add credibility to your work.

References also show how your work contributes to developing ideas in your specific field. Many of your ideas or arguments will be elaborations on work done by others. Referencing helps you show your readers how you have built your own arguments, supporting certain views and ideas and challenging others.

You also need to reference your work to:

- acknowledge the work of others;
- show your reader that you have read up in your field (knowledge display);
- avoid plagiarising the work of others.

Some students find the practice of referencing somehow contradictory. Whereas you have to show a certain degree of originality, you are also supposed to anchor you work on the existing literature. Similarly, you are expected to make a significant contribution of your own but you still have to give credit to the work of others.

On their web-resource page on plagiarism, the Purdue University Online Writing Lab defines the contradictions of academic writing as shown in Figure 10.1.

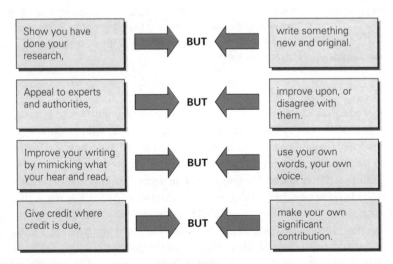

Figure 10.1   Contradictions in referencing

Source: The Purdue University Online Writing Lab.

Contradiction 1: *Show you have done your research, but write something new and original.* One of the reasons why you need to reference your academic work is to show that you have 'done your homework'; that is, you have read the literature connected to the topic you are researching. However, just putting together pieces of what others have said is not enough. You also need to provide something new. This 'something new' needn't be absolutely original; after all 'there is nothing new under the sun'. But you should always try and offer a new approach or a different way of looking at things. This contradiction can be solved by adopting the *'scaffolding technique'* by which you construct new arguments on the basis of previous, more established ones. In the following example the writer has used the scaffolding technique. They have put forward a new argument by referring to what was previously established in relation to reflection:

Established arguments	Reflection has been the focus of several studies which have contributed to making reflection an integral part of the professional nursing practice. In his seminal work, Gibbs (1988) established not only the nature but also the importance of reflection for professional advancement. In a similar manner, Durgahee (1998), elaborating on Gibbs' contribution, examined the application of reflection to nursing. More recently, Johns (2004) has suggested that the main characteristics of reflection include reflexivity, understanding, and empowerment and that these aspects have to be taught to professionals in training. Johns' arguments point to the need for teaching student nurses to reflect and for incorporating reflection activity into the learning process. Introducing students to reflection at an early stage of their training may contribute to a higher degree
New development	of reflexivity in professional practice. This essay will present an argument for the early ...

Contradiction 2: *Appeal to experts and authorities, but improve upon or disagree with them.* Another reason why you need to reference your work is to critically revisit what has been done in the field so as to help it develop. If you merely cite or summarize what has already been said, you are only repeating what is known or given. You also need to improve on what has already been established and, if necessary, be prepared to disagree with it in a critical but constructive manner. This contradiction can be resolved by using the *'critical stance technique'* by means of which you provide a critique of what has been done, highlighting its strengths and pointing to ways in which its weaknesses can be improved. This is illustrated in the following example:

Previous research	Previous studies on geropsychiatric units have focused on the complexity of the care needs of older patients (Brown, 2001), the social and financial difficulties they experience (Allen, 2000) and the specific admission and discharging processes they require (Alexander, 1999). Despite these contributions, research on the needs of the practitioners in this specialized field of nursing care has
New contribution	been scant (Smith *et al.*, 2005). This essay will examine these needs, provide a taxonomy and finally...

Contradiction 3: *Improve your writing by mimicking what you hear and read, but use your own words, your own voice.* There are two sides to this contradiction: mimicking and breaking new ground. When you have to produce a piece of writing you have never produced before, it is always a good idea to look at how more seasoned writers do it. You can look at the way they organize information, what they include in each part of their piece of writing, the language and the style they use. This is mimicking. The other side of this contradiction refers to what we call breaking new ground. When you write, you first try and reach common ground with your readers by using what is known to them, that is, by using the content and the language that you share with your readers. But you definitely have to resort to your own voice when breaking new ground. This contradiction can be resolved by using the '*old and new ground*' technique. For example, you use impersonal structures (e.g. in the passive voice) for what is shared and your own voice (e.g. in the active voice) for what is new. The following example illustrates this technique

Common ground, impersonal structures	It has been argued that for smoking cessation during pregnancy to be successful support to the pregnant smoker has to be structured and sustained (Lumley *et al.*, 2004; Melvin & Gaffney, 2004). Similarly, it has been forcefully argued that programmes of support should consider in-pregnancy as well as postpartum support (Lawrence *et al.*, 2005). This essay argues that unless support for pregnant smokers incorporates strategies by which they learn about the risks of maternal smoking to the fetus and the infant and develop cognitive and behavioural strategies for stopping, it will
New ground, writer's voice	continue making only a marginal impact on smoking cessation during pregnancy.

Contradiction 4: *Give credit where credit is due, but make your own significant contribution.* This final contradiction summarizes the preceding ones. It refers to the fact that you must reference when you are borrowing other people's ideas and/or words but you can't merely produce a summary of what has been previously done or said. You also need to help advance the field by making a new and significant contribution or by presenting a new approach to an already established topic.

Activity 10.2

Read the following texts and decide what technique has been used to develop them.

Text 1

Vaginal examination on admission and during labour is probably one of the most common procedures performed by midwives. These examinations have been studied in terms of when they should be performed and how frequently (Gibb, 1991; Lefeber & Voorhoeve, 1998). There has been, however, a noticeable paucity in studies examining women's feelings and experiences of vaginal examinations (Lai & Levy, 2002). This critique analyses...

Text 2

Much has been written about the psychological and emotional effects of gynaecological cancer on women. Effects on altered fertility and sexual dysfunction (Anderson *et al.*, 1992; Cull *et al.*, 1993) have long been recognised in the literature. The psychological and emotional effects on the male partners of women with gynaecological cancer have however received very little attention (Maughan *et al.*, 2002). This essay explores the emotional effects of male partners and ...

Answers See suggested answers on page 201.

● Referencing systems

Now that we have discussed the reasons for referencing, let us have a look at the mechanics of referencing. There are two types of referencing systems used:

- author-date systems (e.g. Harvard system and APA);
- numerical systems (e.g. Chicago and Vancouver systems).

An example following an author-date system would look like this:

Text Reflection has proved essential for the professional development of nurses (Gibbs, 1988).

List of references	Gibbs, G. (1988) *Learning by Doing. A guide to teaching and learning methods*. Further Education Unit. Oxford: Oxford Polytechnic.

The same example but following a numerical system would look like this:

Text	Reflection has proved essential for the professional development of nurses [1].

List of references	[1] Gibbs, G. (1988) *Learning by Doing. A guide to teaching and learning methods*. Further Education Unit. Oxford: Oxford Polytechnic.

In author-date systems, sources in the list of references are organized alphabetically, while in numerical systems they are organized numerically, in the order they appeared in the text.

There are two basic ways of using references in your texts:

- in-text citation;
- quotation.

In-text citation is used when you borrow somebody else's ideas only, not their words. In-text citation acknowledges the source of ideas you are writing about in your own words. You can do this by:

- adding references in brackets at the end of your own idea (e.g. Reflection has been identified as an extremely useful skill for nurses (Durgahee, 1996; Johns, 1996; Mountford and Rogers, 1996); or
- mentioning the author(s) and paraphrasing their ideas in your own words (e.g. Allen (1990) suggests that patients ...).

It is important to notice that there is a slight difference in emphasis between these two ways of using in-text citations. In the first case, where you use parenthetical references, the emphasis is on the ideas or contributions made by the author or authors. In the second, you emphasize the author's or authors' importance. This difference in emphasis is important as you may sometimes need to specify the contribution made to the field by a specific person. For example, in most sources about reflection you will come across 'Gibbs (1988)' as his name is associated with the development of reflective practice in nursing.

When you borrow not only other people's ideas – acknowledged by citation – but also their words, you are using quotation. Quoted text must be included between quotation marks ('like this text') to indicate these are the exact words of the original text. Quotation marks also serve the purpose of separating your own words from those of other people. This is a basic tool to help you avoid plagiarism (also see Chapter 9).

In the case of quotations, you must provide:

- the surname(s) of the author(s);
- the year of the publication; and
- the page number(s) of the original text.

In summary, you need to reference when you:

- borrow ideas or information from other sources;
- quote somebody's words and ideas exactly as they were in the original text;
- paraphrase somebody's ideas in your own words;
- summarize somebody's ideas in your own words;
- reproduce a graph, table or diagram from other sources.

The way in which you organize these pieces of information will vary depending on the referencing system you need to follow. In nursing and midwifery, the most commonly used systems of referencing are the Harvard system and the American Psychological Association (APA) style. The Vancouver system is also used though less commonly. We will examine these three systems in more detail in the next sections.

● The Harvard system

The Harvard system is a popular method of referencing in higher education. It is in fact the most commonly used system in nursing and midwifery studies, and in the following tables you will find the most common conventions for referencing sources following the Harvard system. Conventions for in-text citations and quotations are listed in Tables 10.1 and 10.2, while conventions for lists of references are given in Table 10.3 on page 164.

Convention	Avoid	Example
In-text citations should include the author's or authors' surnames (up to 3 authors), followed by the year of publication.	Using first names or first-name initials.	This has been identified as a central issue in contemporary health care (Perry, 2004).
Use ampersand (&) for sources by more than one author.	Using ampersand in direct quotes.	The potential causes of maternal postnatal concern and distress have been examined from different perspectives (Littlewood & McHugh, 1997).
When paraphrasing other people's ideas, use their surname(s), followed by the year of publication in round brackets.	Using ampersand (&) when the author(s) are not within brackets.	Potter and Perry (2004) have identified it as a central issue in contemporary health care.
When you cite more than one source, you can organize them in either alphabetical or chronological order.	Mixing both styles in the same text and using a comma between surname(s) and date.	This view has been supported by many prac-titioners (Allen, 2002; Brown, 2001; Roberts, 2000). This view has been supported by many practitioners (Roberts, 2000; Brown, 2001; Allen, 2002).
Use the phrase 'as cited in' followed by the source details when you are quoting something already quoted in your source. Include both sources in the list of references.	Quoting the secondary source as if you had read it.	Smith (1999, as cited in Clark, 2004, p. 121) supported the idea of a new approach to nurse education which would include a strong reflective element.
Use 'et al.' ('and others') for a source that has more than 3 authors. Use *italics* for this abbreviation.	Using a full stop after 'et'. It's a complete word. It is Latin for 'and'.	New approaches to woman care tend to place both the woman and the midwife at the centre of the care (Pairman *et al.*, 2006).

Table 10.1 Conventions for in-text citations using the Harvard system

Convention	Avoid	Example
Use page numbers **only** if you reproduce (e.g. quote, paraphrase, or summarize) information from another source.	Using a colon between year and page. Instead use a comma after the year and 'p.' before the page number. In case of two or more pages, use 'pp.'	However, as Page (2000, p. 10) points out 'women having home births are well educated and healthy, and this may be a major factor influencing the outcomes of such studies.'
Quotations that are longer than 2 or 3 lines should be separated from the main text, indented and single spaced and put into smaller font.	Using quotation marks for longer quotes.	Your text your text your text your text your text Long quote long quote long quote long quote long quote Your text your text your text your text.
Quotations from internet resources with no pagination should mention the paragraph number or line in the original text.	Paginating the web-based source yourself. Using the URL of the page in your text.	Stark (2004, line 34) claims that 'these areas of concern have tended to go unnoticed in most research to date'.
If no date is given in the source (e.g. a pamphlet), use the abbreviation 'n.d.' (no date).		This is a crucial step in educating the new mother (Enfield Health Centre n.d.).
Use the title of a source if you can't identify its author(s). This also applies to work published by a group organization.	Using 'anonymous' for newspapers or other popular sources.	The health and well-being of the ageing population is a growing concern that requires intelligent and innovative responses (*Our health, our care, our say*, DoH 2006).
For an article without an author (e.g. newspaper), use the name of the publication instead.		Overseas nurses in the UK have encountered problems for being promoted to better, more challenging positions (*The Guardian* 2005).

Table 10.2 Conventions for quotations using the Harvard system

Activity 10.3

Based on what you have learnt about in-text citations and quotations following the Harvard system, read this text and identify what is wrong with each reference.

Dual diagnosis specialists are becoming increasingly aware of the need to develop a treatment model that addresses the challenges posed by clients with severe mental health problems and a history of misuse substances (Philips P. & Joanne Labrow, 1998). There are a few intervention programmes to treat clients with a dual diagnosis. However, they are relatively new and have not been objectively evaluated for their effectiveness (Rassool, 2001, pp.110). In some countries, increasing attention to these issues is being paid and, as a result, several integrated approach treatment programmes have been set up. These involve specialized multidisciplinary teams, working to address the unmet needs of clients (www.mind.org.uk). This essay will briefly describe the existing models, and thoroughly examine their value. Against this background, the essay will evaluate the potentials of the new programmes in the light of the results obtained in their implementation.

Answers See suggested answers on page 202.

● The American Psychological Association (APA) Style

The APA style is also an author-date system sometimes recommended by some nursing and midwifery lecturers. However, it is more common in publications such as professional journals.

In Tables 10.4 and 10.5 you will find the most common conventions for referencing sources following the APA style that differ from the ones given for the Harvard style.

Convention	Avoid	Example
References should be alphabetically organized.	Using bullets or numbers for the sources in your list.	Courtenay, M. 2002. .... Godin, P. 2003a. .... Godin, P. 2003b. ... Warne, T. and S. McAndrew. 2004....
Use *italics* for the title of books and name of journals. Capitalize only their first word.	Using italics for the title of chapters in books and articles in journals.	Warne, T. and S. McAndrew. 2004. *Using patient experience in nurse education*. Basingstoke: Palgrave.
The author's surname should be followed by a comma and the author's name initial or initials, followed by the year of publication.	Using brackets for the year of publication.	Jasper, M. 2003. *Beginning reflective practice: Foundations in nursing and health care*. Cheltenham: Nelson Thornes.
Titles of chapters and articles should be enclosed in single quotes and capitalized only in their first word. Page numbers should also be given.	Using double quotation marks ("text").	Courtenay, M. 2002. 'Movement and mobility' in R. Hogston and P. M. Simpson (eds): *Foundations of nursing practice*, 262–285. Basingstoke: Palgrave.
Include the edition of a book only if it is **not** the first.	Using 'ed' to abbreviate edition. Use 'edn' instead. Sometimes 'e' is used as in '2e' (second edition), but this has not become an established convention yet.	Johnson, T. and W. Taylor. 2005. *Skills for midwifery practice*. Second edn. London: Churchill Livingstone.

Convention	Avoid	Example
Internet resources (e.g. webpages) should contain the complete URL (uniform resource locator) and the date it was last accessed.		'Standards of proficiency for nurse and midwife prescribers'. 2005. NMC. Available at http://www.nmc-uk.org/ aFrameDisplay.aspx? DocumentID=1645, accessed: 02.06.06.
Use letters (a, b, c) after the year for multiple publications by the same author(s) in the same year.		Godin, P. 2003a. 'Class inequalities in mental health nursing' in M. Miers (ed.): *Class inequalities and nursing practice*, 125–143. Basingstoke: Palgrave. Godin, P. 2003b. 'The frontline workforce of community mental health care' in B. Hannigan and M. Coffey (eds): *The handbook of community mental health nursing*, London: Routledge. Godin, P. 2003c. 'Be very afraid', *Mental health nursing*, 23(3) pp. 12–13.
Include the editor's or editors' names in edited collections. Notice that in this case the order of the editor's or editors' surname and name initials is reversed.	Using '(ed.)' for volumes that have been edited by more than one editor. Use '(eds)' instead.	Courtenay, M. 2002. 'Movement and mobility' in R. Hogston and P. M. Simpson (eds): *Foundations of nursing practice*, 262–285. Basingstoke: Palgrave.

Table 10.3 Conventions for lists of references using the Harvard system

Convention	Avoid	Example
In-text citations should include the author's or authors' surnames (up to 3), followed by a comma, followed by the year of publication.	Using first names or first names initials.	This has been identified as a central issue in contemporary health care (Potter & Perry, 2004).
When you cite more than one source, organize them alphabetically and separate them with a semi-colon.		This view has been supported by many practitioners (Allen, 2002; Brown, 2001; Roberts, 2000).
The first time you use a source with more than 3 authors, use all surnames. Use the first author's surname followed by 'et al.' ('and others') for subsequent citations of the source. Use *italics* for this abbreviation.	Using a full stop after 'et'.	Care for the pregnant woman has been a crucial issue in midwifery (Pairman, Pincombe, Thorogood & Tracy, 2006). New approaches to woman care tend to place both the woman and the midwife at the centre of the care (Pairman *et al.*, 2006).
Use ampersand (&) for more than one author in in-text citation	Using ampersand (&) when the author(s) are not within brackets	The potential causes of maternal postnatal concern and distress have been examined from different perspectives (Littlewood & McHugh, 1997).

Table 10.4   Conventions for in-text citations and quotations using the APA style

● The Vancouver system

The Vancouver system is a numerical system in which a number is assigned to each reference as it appears in the text. This number becomes the 'unique identifier' of that reference and is used each time that reference is cited. In other words, the first reference you cite will be numbered 1 in the text, and

Convention	Avoid	Example
The author's surname should be followed by a comma and the author's name initial or initials, followed by the year of publication between round brackets.		Jasper, M. (2003). *Beginning reflective practice: Foundations in nursing and health care*. Cheltenham: Nelson Thornes.
Titles of book chapters should NOT be enclosed in quotes and should be capitalized only in their first word. Page numbers should appear in round brackets.		Courtenay, M. 2002. Movement and mobility, in R. Hogston and P. M. Simpson (eds), *Foundations of nursing practice* (pp. 262–285). Basingstoke: Palgrave.
For journal articles, use italics for the name of the journal, followed by a comma, followed by the issue number, followed by a comma and the page numbers.	Using the abbreviation 'pp.' for the page numbers, and round brackets.	Fine, M. A. & Kurdek, L. A. (1993). Reflections on determining authorship credit and authorship order on faculty-student collaborations. *American Psychologist*, 48, 1141–1147.

Table 10.5   Conventions for lists of references using the APA style

Activity 10.4

Based on what you have learnt about lists of references following the APA style, read this text and spot any errors or omissions.

Courtenay, M. 2002. Movement and mobility in R. Hogston and P. M. Simpson (eds): *Foundations of nursing practice*, 262-285. Basingstoke: Palgrave.

Johnson, T and W. Taylor. (2005). *Skills for midwifery practice*. Second edn. London: Churchill Livingstone.

Jasper, M. (2003). *Beginning reflective practice: Foundations in nursing and health care*. Cheltenham: Nelson Thornes.

Savage, T. A. (2005). How do we handle conflicts with parents over unsafe oral feedings? *Rehabilitation Nursing*, 30, (pp. 7–8).

Answers   See suggested answers on page 202.

Convention	Example
Numbers are inserted to the right of commas and full stops, and to the left of colons and semi-colons.	Using first names or first name initials. This has been identified as a central issue in contemporary health care. (1)
Multiple sources can be listed at a single reference point. The numbers are then separated by commas and consecutive numbers are joined with a hyphen.	The potential causes of maternal post natal concern and distress have been examined from different perspectives. (2–6, 11, 21)

Table 10.6　Main in-text citation conventions for the Vancouver system

the second reference you cite will be numbered 2. When you cite reference number 1 again, you will cite it using the number 1. Even when the name of the author appears in your text, it should be followed by the number of the reference.

Let us look at an example. This same example appeared on page 124 but following the Harvard system of referencing. You may then wish to compare both examples and see how a numerical and an author-date system differ. The main conventions for in-text citations, quotations and references are listed in Tables 10.6–10.8.

Convention	Example
Use double quotation marks to enclose a direct quotation.	However, as Page points out "women having home births are well educated and healthy, and this may be a major factor influencing the outcomes of such studies." (3)
Quotations that are longer than 2 or 3 lines should be separated from the main text, indented and single spaced and put into smaller font.	Your text your text your text your text your text (4) 　　Long quote long quote long quote long quote long quote Your text your text your text your text.

Table 10.7　Main quotation conventions for the Vancouver system

Convention	Example
The reference list is arranged numerically in the order in which references are cited in the text.	(1) Courtenay M. ... (2) Godin P. ... (3) Warne T. and S. McAndrew ... (4) Allen P. ...
Use normal font for the title of books and name of journals. Capitalize only their first word and proper names.	Warne T. and S. McAndrew. Using patient experience in nurse education. Basingstoke: Palgrave; 2004.
The author's surname should be followed by the author's name initial or initials with no punctuation separating them. A full stop should follow.	Jasper M.
Author's names should be followed by the title of book or journal article. A full stop should follow.	Beginning reflective practice: Foundations in nursing and health care.
The title of the book should be followed by the place of publication, followed by a colon, and then followed by the publishing house. A semi-colon should follow. Finally the year of publication should be added.	Cheltenham: Nelson Thornes; 2003.
In the case of a journal article, the title of the article should be followed by the abbreviated name of the journal, followed by the year of publication, followed by a semi-colon, followed by the volume and issue number, followed by a colon, followed by the page numbers.	Wharton N. Health and safety in outdoor activity centres. J Adventure Ed Outdoor Lead. 1996;12(4):8–9.
Journal titles are abbreviated. A list of abbreviations for the titles is available from PubMed at http://www.ncbi.nih.gov/entrez/query.fcgi. To view the abbreviated form of a journal title, click on "Journals Database" and then enter the full journal title.	Some examples of journal abbreviations: Pract Midwife.: The Practising Midwife Nurs Stand.: Nursing Standard Nurs Ethics.: Nursing Ethics Community Pract.: Community Practitioner J Adv Nurs.: Journal of Advanced Nursing

Table 10.8   List of reference conventions for the Vancouver system

The differences seen are not explainable by disappointment with the care-giver assignment. Staniszewska and Ahmed (1) point out that patients' expectations are influenced by their awareness of what they realistically expect. Evaluation of a service is also influenced by beliefs about the duty the service owes the client and whether or not there were circumstances outside the service's control that affected the care (2). If expectations are a determinant of satisfaction with care, there is then less difference between the satisfaction scores of the two groups since women have different expectations for doctors than they do for midwives.

(Adapted from Harvey *et al.*, 2002: 266)

● Bibliographic software programmes

Bibliographic software programmes are packages that can help you organize your references. They are relatively easy to use and more and more universities are adopting them. They contain most referencing styles (both author-date and numerical systems) and you can change styles once you have created your own library of references.

In this section, you will find a short description and some examples of two of these software programmes: EndNote and RefWorks.

EndNote

EndNote is a tool designed to help you manage your references, among other things. (A free trial of EndNote can be downloaded from http://www.endnote.com/). With EndNote you can:

- Search bibliographic databases on the Internet;
- Organize references and images in a database;
- Create your own library of references;
- Add a new reference, or change it or delete it;
- Construct your paper with built-in manuscript templates;
- Watch the bibliography and figure list appear as you write.

Because EndNote works in a Windows environment, it will be easy for you to use it if you are familiar with any Windows word processor.

Adding a new reference is done by type (e.g. journal article, book, conference proceedings, etc.) and you do not need to worry about formatting (capitals, font type, etc.) as EndNote will do it for you according to the style you select. The template for adding new data, called a blank data-entry screen, is

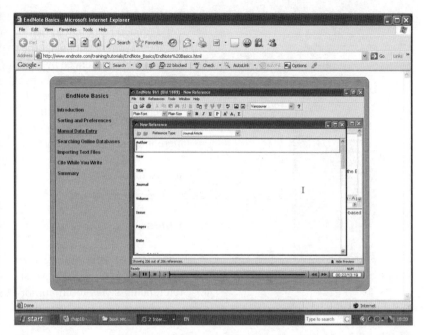

Figure 10.2 An EndNote blank data entry screen

shown in Figure 10.2. The window for managing the data you entered should look like Figure 10.3.

Once you have created your own library using the form shown above, you can manage the references in it. As Figure 10.3 illustrates, in the managing data window you can see the list of references in the library you have created. A reference can be highlighted to see the complete notes you made for it, and the list can be displayed by either author, year or title.

Another very interesting facility that EndNote offers is the possibility of inserting references in your paper as you write. This facility is called 'cite while you write' (CWYW). For this, you need to access EndNote from the 'Tools' dropdown menu of your word processor, that enables you to use EndNote within your word processor document. You will also have an EndNote toolbar from which you can find a reference you need, insert it into your document and choose the style you need your references to observe. EndNote includes more than 1,300 bibliographic styles. An EndNote screen for 'cite while you write' should look like Figure 10.4.

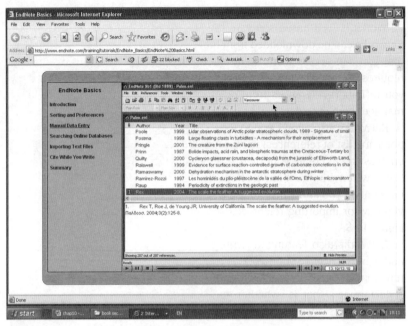

Figure 10.3 An EndNote managing data window

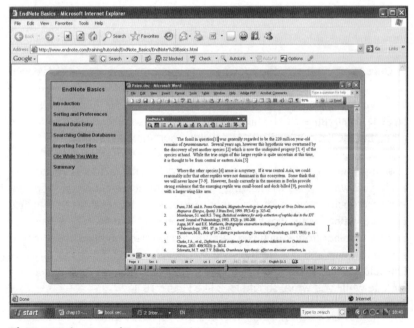

Figure 10.4 An EndNote CWYW screen

RefWorks

RefWorks is web-based software to manage bibliographies. (A free trial of Refworks can be downloaded from http://www.refworks.com/). This means that you can access it from any internet-connected computer or laptop; it requires no special software and is automatically upgraded. RefWorks allows you to import references from different sources, organize them and easily manage them in folders.

RefWorks also allows you to format your references (for both in-text citations and list of references) in more than 500 styles. Added to this, RefWorks enables you to create your own style of referencing. The software works in a Windows environment and it should be very simple for you to become familiar with it if you know how to use a Windows word processor. The RefWorks window for importing references should look like the screenshot shown in Figure 10.5.

RefWorks also features a 'write and cite' function that you can use for adding references to your work as you write. This is simply done by using the function 'inserting' in your word processor. A window for defining the output style format – that is, whether you want to use the Harvard or the APA system, for instance – looks as shown in Figure 10.6.

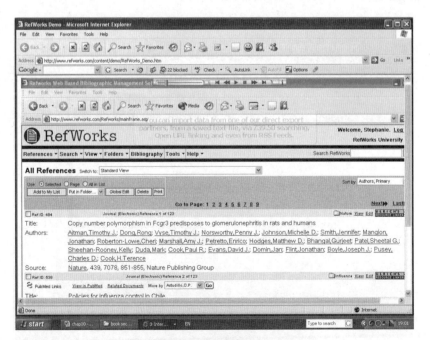

Figure 10.5   Importing references with RefWorks

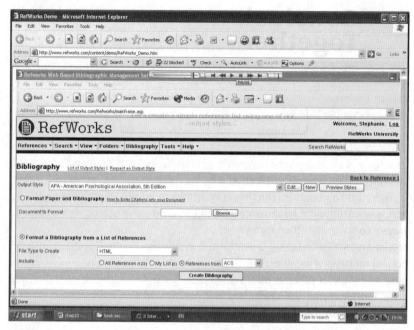

Figure 10.6 Defining the output style in Refworks

Revising the objectives of this chapter

Tick those objectives you feel you have achieved and review those you have not yet managed to accomplish. Then complete the Achievement Chart at the back of the book.

In this chapter, you have learnt to:

☐ recognize the basic principles for referencing

☐ identify the main referencing conventions of the Harvard, the APA and the Vancouver systems

☐ recognize the basic uses of bibliographic software programmes

11 Conclusion: Putting it all Together

Like any other type of writing, academic writing is best approached as a **process** and a **product**. The process starts with an examination of the question your assignment has to answer and a consideration of the most effective ways to answer it. It then moves on to gathering relevant information and to organizing and structuring this information into blocks. But more often than not, when structuring information you will probably need to go back to planning so as to reorganize information in the most effective way. Once you have written your first draft, you will need to become an editor of your product. Editing your work requires a combination of macro abilities that you use in the writing process to look at the organization and structuring of information, and micro skills that you need to look at sentence structure and punctuation, for instance.

The chapters in the book have been arranged in three parts which examine both the process and the product of writing. In the first part, you covered **the essentials of academic writing**: examining assignment questions, gathering information, and organizing and structuring the information into paragraphs, and paragraphs into essays. You also explored the differences between descriptive and argumentative writing, and examined typical genres that require these types of writing: the care critique, the journal article review and the argumentative essay. You finally analysed two essential processes that form the basis for many of these academic genres: reflection and critical thinking.

In the second part of the book you learnt **how to write specific genres** in nursing and midwifery. The first chapter in this part elaborated on the foundations laid in the previous part and it examined how to write a reflective essay. Then you moved on to analyse a more analytic genre: the care critique. You explored planning and organizing principles in writing a care critique, and learnt to structure it more effectively as well as to make sensible recommendations. Next, you learnt how to write argumentative texts and looked at three essential elements in argumentation: the strength of an argument, its structure and its language. The last chapter in this second part introduced you to the basics of writing other typical genres in nursing and midwifery: action plans, care plans, portfolios, reports, and research proposals. It also showed the preliminary steps you need to take when preparing to write your undergraduate dissertation.

The first two parts dealt with academic writing as a process. The last section approached writing as a product, giving you the basic tools to become the editor of your own work. In this last part, you learnt to **work with texts**. You learnt how to add variety to your texts, how to make them more cohesive and you looked into what we call 'good writing style'. Coupled with this, in this part you dealt with plagiarism and learnt how to reference sources correctly following an author–date or a numerical referencing system.

It is important for you to see writing as both a **process** and a **product**. As a process, writing means drafting and redrafting. Even the most accomplished writers need to draft and redraft, moving from planning to structuring, only to go back to planning again. As a product, you need to learn to become an editor of your own work, distancing yourself from it and using the marking criteria for the assignment you're writing to make sure your 'product' meets the demands of the task at hand. To this end, you can use the different checklists in the chapters of this book to help you edit your work. More importantly, use the book checklists as the basis on which to design your own.

We started this book with the idea that academic writing is one of the most difficult tasks we encounter when we start university. As with all other academic tasks, academic writing is a skill that can be learnt and perfected with dedication and practice. I hope that now that you have reached the end of the book you will feel more confident about writing your assignments. You have covered all the necessary theoretical background you need to know to be able to write effectively, and you have also done exercises which have illustrated the main theoretical principles. Now you are ready to put it all together; to put theory into practice!

● Achievement chart

Use the following chart to plot your achievements. If you have not achieved an objective (**✗**) or you are not sure about it (**?**), plan some action that will contribute to its achievemnt, for example revise the corresponding section in the book or ask your personal or support tutor for guidance.

ACHIEVEMENT CHART

Unit (chapter)	Objectives (by chapter section)	Achieved ✔/✗/?	Action to take
1	▲ Recognize the five basic principles of academic writing.		
	▲ Identify the three elements in essay questions and follow marking criteria.		
	▲ Understand gathering, organizing and structuring information.		
	▲ Reproduce the generic structure of academic texts.		
	▲ Identify main problems with sentence fragments, cohesion, dangling modifiers and punctuation.		
2	▲ Recognize the difference between description and argumentation.		
	▲ Identify the main academic genres in nursing and midwifery.		

© Julio Gimenez (2007), *Writing for Nursing and Midwifery Students*, Palgrave Macmillan Ltd.

Unit (chapter)	Objectives (by chapter section)	Achieved ✔/✗/?	Action to take
	▶ Understand the purpose and the structure of these academic genres.		
	▶ Identify main language items used in descriptive and critical writing.		
3	▶ Recognize the nature and stages of the reflective process.		
	▶ Identify different critical thinking processes.		
	▶ Understand the principles of critical evaluation of evidence.		
	▶ Identify key language items used in reflective and critical writing.		
4	▶ Plan a reflective essay appropriately.		
	▶ Identify an effective way of introducing reflective essays.		
	▶ Recognize the structure of body paragraphs to support introductions.		

Unit (chapter)	Objectives (by chapter section)	Achieved ✔/✗/?	Action to take
	▲ Recognize ways of producing an effective conclusion.		
	▲ Identify the style of the reflective essay.		
5	▲ Plan and organize the care critique effectively.		
	▲ Structure the main sections of the care critique.		
	▲ Provide effective conclusions and make sensible recommendations.		
6	▲ Recognize the difference between opinion and argumentation.		
	▲ Identify the strength of an argument.		
	▲ Structure arguments effectively.		
	▲ Identify main language items used in argumentative writing.		

© Julio Gimenez (2007), *Writing for Nursing and Midwifery Students*, Palgrave Macmillan Ltd.

Unit (chapter)	Objectives (by chapter section)	Achieved ✔/✗/?	Action to take
7	▲ Write actions plans.		
	▲ Write care plans.		
	▲ Prepare, write and choose an appropriate format for portfolios.		
	▲ Produce reports.		
	▲ Identify effective ways of producing research and dissertation proposals.		
	▲ Plan to start writing your dissertation.		
8	▲ Recognize different ways of adding variety to your texts.		
	▲ Identify different sentence openers.		
	▲ Use cohesive devices to support textual variety.		
	▲ Recognize different structural elements used for adding variety between parts of a text.		

Unit (chapter)	Objectives (by chapter section)	Achieved ✔/✗/?	Action to take
9	▲ Recognize what constitutes plagiarism and what does not.		
	▲ Deal with definitions and concepts already well-established in your field.		
	▲ Paraphrase other people's ideas and words without plagiarizing.		
10	▲ Recognize the basic principles of referencing.		
	▲ Identify the main referencing conventions of the Harvard system.		
	▲ Identify the main referencing conventions of the APA system.		
	▲ Identify the main referencing conventions of the Vancouver system.		
	▲ be familiar with bibliographic software programmes.		

© Julio Gimenez (2007), *Writing for Nursing and Midwifery Students*, Palgrave Macmillan Ltd.

Glossary of Key Terms

Note: Numbers in brackets indicate the chapter which deals with the word/phrase being defined.

A

Argumentative writing: Writing that aims at persuading the reader about the validity, importance or significance of a point made or stance taken by the writer. It uses evidence to support the claims made and usually makes recommendations. (**2**)

Articles: There are three articles in English: 'a' and 'an' (indefinite articles) and 'the' (definite article). (**7**)

Article review: A piece of writing that evaluates an article published in an academic or professional journal. (**2**)

Assessment/ marking criteria: A set of principles used to judge the value and contribution of a written piece. In academic writing the assessment or marking criteria for an assignment normally accompany the instructions for it. (**1**) (**7**)

B

Bibliographic references: name of the author, title, name of publication, and other bibliographical details. (**2**)

Bibliography: The list of sources that have been consulted or used in preparation of an academic document. This is presented at the end of an academic document and organized alphabetically. (Cf. list of references) (**1**)

C

Care critique: A systematic, critical and impersonal analysis of the care provided to a patient. A care critique discusses the validity and evaluates the worth of the care. (**2**)

Claim: Something that is believed to be true and that is supported by evidence. (**6**)

Cohesion: What holds texts together. Cohesion is normally achieved by using connectives, related words or logical transitions. See also 'Logical relationships' (**1**)

Critical analysis: Systematic, logical and impersonal examination of the contents included, the claims made and the sources of evidence used in an argument. (**2**)

Critical skills: Sets of abilities needed to examine and evaluate the worth and contribution of an argument, a piece of writing, etc. (**7**)

E

Evidence-based: Evidence-based clinical or academic practice emphasizes the examination of evidence from research or reflection upon clinical experience as the basis for decision-making. It de-emphasizes intuition, and unsystematic experience, and requires skills such as literature searching, and critical evaluation of sources. (**1**)

F

Font size: The size of the font used in a computer word processor and measured in points. In academic documents, the common size is 11 or 12 points. (**1**)

Font style: The type of font used in a computer word processor. In academic documents, the common font styles are Arial and Times New Roman. Fanciful fonts are normally avoided. (**1**)

G

Genres: The word genre comes from the French (originally Latin) word for 'kind' or 'class'. Genres can be said to constitute particular conventions of content and/or form (including structure and style). These conventions are shared by all the texts that belong to the same 'class' or genre. Thus, all reflective essays, for example, will share certain conventions as to content and form. (**2**)

Generic genre: A genre that can be used as the basis for producing other associated genres. For example, the academic essay can be said to be a generic genre on which the reflective essay can be structured. (**2**)

Generic functions: The function that a part of a genre is supposed to fulfil. For example, one generic function that introductions are supposed to have is 'stating the purpose of the text'. (**5**)

L

List of references: List of all the sources cited in a text. The list is presented at the end of an academic document and organized alphabetically. (**1**)

Logical relationships: Relationships between the ideas in a text that are emphasized by the use of 'connectives'. See also 'Cohesion'. (**2**) (**8**)

N

Narrow down: To focus on main points by selection or reducing them in number. (**1**)

O

Outline: Schematic representation or plan for producing a piece of writing. (**4**)

P

Paragraph: A group of related (in topic and focus) sentences that makes complete sense in its own. Paragraphs may be short or long, the important thing about paragraphs is that they develop only one central idea. (**1**)

Paragraphing: Arranging and structuring information into paragraphs. (**1**)

Paraphrasing: Expressing the same ideas and content of an original text, but using different words and structural elements. (**9**)

Parentheses: ( ) Punctuation marks used to add extra, parenthetical information which is not necessary to understand the main/central idea being expressed. E.g. 'In this format, the items are arranged in the order specified above (with exception for specialized entries).' (**1**)

Persuasive reasoning: Argumentative writing that aims at convincing or persuading the readers. (**2**).

Plagiarism: Intellectual dishonesty by which someone claims other people's ideas or texts are their own. Plagiarism is usually the result of ignorance or cultural differences. Some students ignore the rules for citation and quotation that are regulated by different referencing systems. In some cultures, 'copying' other people's intellectual property may be considered a 'complement'. (**9**)

Punctuation marks: Punctuation marks are used to signal pause, emphasis, expansion or clarification. The most frequently used punctuation marks are the apostrophe, colon, comma, dash, hyphen, parentheses, quotation marks, and semicolon. (**1**)

Q

Question words: Words used to ask questions, sometimes called 'wh' words: what, where, when, why, who. But also notice: how, how often, how long. (**1**)

R

Rationale: The reasons that explain why a particular decision has been made, a course of action followed, etc. (**1**)

Referencing: A system of rules to cite and quote other people's intellectual property which helps writers to avoid committing plagiarism. There are a number of systems, the most frequent being The Harvard System, the American Psychology Association (APA) system and the Modern Language Association (MLA) system. (**10**)

Reflection: The process by which a past event or occurrence is revisited to evaluate, from the present perspective, what happened and how its negative effects can be avoided in the future. (**3**)

Rephrase: Say something again by using different words. See also 'Paraphrase' (**1**)

S

Signpost: A word, phrase or sentence that is used to indicate the direction an argument or idea will take or follow. (**1**)

Stance: Position that the writer of a text adopts in relation to the text he/she is producing. Stance is normally created by the use of linguistic devices such as 'modal verbs', and 'adverbs'. (**2**)

Supporting evidence: Evidence or practice-based examples used to support a claim made. (**1**)

T

Text flow: The way ideas connect with one another in a text. The logical flow between the ideas in a text is reinforced by formal elements such as connectives, and lexis. See also 'Cohesion'. (**1**)

Tone down: Make the claims made less comprehensive, extreme or offensive. (**6**)

Transitions/transition markers: A word, phrase or sentence used to mark the transition between ideas or paragraphs in a text. Transition markers are used to reinforce the flow between parts of a text or between texts. (**3**) (**4**)

Further Readings and Resources

This list indicates books and websites you can turn to if you want to expand on any of the main topics in this text.

Critical thinking

Cottrell, Stella (2005) *Critical Thinking Skills. Developing Effective Analysis and Argument*. Basingstoke: Palgrave Macmillan.

Milan, Deanne (2006) *Developing Critical Reading Skills*, 7th edn. New York: McGraw-Hill.

Van Den Brinkbudgen, Roy (2000) *Critical Thinking for Students: Learn the Skills of Critical Assessment and Effective Argument*, 3rd edn. Oxford: How to Books.

Resources
Palgrave critical /analytical thinking skills
   http://www.palgrave.com/skills4study/html/studyskills/critical.htm

Plagiarism

Johns, Julia and Sarah Keller (2005) *Cite It Right: The SourceAid Guide to Citation, Research, and Avoiding Plagiarism*. Boston, MA: SourceAid, LLC.

Pears, Richard and Graham Shields (2005) *Cite Them Right: The Essential Guide to Referencing and Plagiarism*. Newcastle upon Tyne: Pear Tree Books.

Punctuation

Peck, John and Martin Coyle (1999) *The Student's Guide to Writing. Grammar, Punctuation and Spelling*. Basingstoke: Palgrave Macmillan.

Peck, John and Martin Coyle (2005) *Write it Right. A Handbook for Students*. Basingstoke: Palgrave Macmillan.

Resources
University of Ottawa Punctuation Web-page
  http://www.uottawa.ca/academic/arts/writcent/hypergrammar/punct.
  html

Referencing
Greetham, Bryan (2001) *How to Write Better Essays*. Basingstoke: Palgrave
  Macmillan.

Working with tables, charts and graphs
Etherington, Sue (2002) *Tables, Charts and Graphs*. Essential computers
  series. London: Dorling Kindersley Publishers Ltd.
Smyth, T.R. (2004) *The Principles of Writing in Psychology*. Basingstoke:
  Palgrave Macmillan.

Suggested Answers to Activities

Chapter 1

Activity 1.1

The table below lists the verbs you will see most often used in essay questions. Write the meaning of each verb in your own words. You do not need to provide complete sentences; key words will do. Use a dictionary if you are not sure of the meanings. 'Argue' and 'discuss' have been done for you as examples.

Verb	Definition	Additional information
Analyse	*To examine the structure or components of something to explain it.*	*To separate into parts.*
Argue	To give reasons why something is right or wrong, true or untrue.	To persuade people.
Classify	*To sort into groups.*	*According to features.*
Demonstrate	*To show what something is like, or how it works.*	*Using evidence.*
Differentiate	*To show main differences between things.*	Key features or *qualities.*
Discuss	To examine in detail, showing the different opinions or ideas about something.	Frequently confused with 'argue', but a more balanced response is required in 'discuss'.

Evaluate	To calculate or judge the value of something.	It may require personal views.
Examine	To consider something carefully.	Considering its structure, components, etc.
Explain	To give the reasons why something is what it is, or happens the way it does.	To get a better understanding of it.
Identify	To spot something and be able to say what it is.	Main features or qualities.
Outline	To give a description of main features or issues.	Brief.
Produce	To show something for examination.	

Activity 1.2

How would you organize and structure them to write an essay on this question?
Here is one possibility. There may be others, but it's important that you realize the list presents positive as well as negative aspects of communication in nursing.

The importance of effective communication in nursing

Positive
- Communication as a therapeutic space
- Collaboration and negotiation skills with clients and families
- Facilitating empathy

Negative
- Common barriers to effective communication
- Dealing with aggression

Activity 1.3

The paragraph has five sentences. Can you identify

1 the sentence that introduces the general idea of the text (**topic**)?
   Nurses can work in many health care settings, which gives them the opportunity to gain experience in all aspects of caring for clients and their families.

2 another sentence that provides the focus/point of view of the topic (**focus**)?
   Nurses can thus build their professional career in many different ways.

3 the examples that develop/support the focus (**examples/ evidence**)?
   They may choose to become clinical specialists or consultant nurses, or they can opt for managerial positions as a head of nursing services or supervisor of other nurses. Some may prefer to pursue an academic career in education and research.

4 the sentence that brings the text to an end (**conclusion**)?
   These are just a few examples of the opportunities that nurses currently have to develop their professional interests.

Chapter 2

Activity 2.1

What does providing care for the critically ill patient involve? Discuss.

Introduction 1
It provides a good start with a clear topic and focus. However, it doesn't include much more than that. It doesn't say how they essay will be developed, and it is very difficult to anticipate what you will find in it.

Analyse the role of reassurance in nursing care.

Introduction 2
It is a very good start of an introduction. It clearly identifies the topic and the focus. It organizes information from general to specific and provides enough information to understand the point it is trying to make. It also includes a short description of what the essay will do. It is, however, a bit incomplete as it does not mention everything the essay will do, which you expect after the connective 'first'.

Evaluate the value of models for treating dual diagnosis clients.

Introduction 3
This is a very good and complete introduction. It has a clear topic and focus. It includes enough information for the reader to know what it is going to be about. It also states how the essay will go about developing its topic and its focus.

Activity 2.2

This is a very effective outline. It covers all points related to the essay question and shows that the writer is aware of the marking criteria, especially criteria 2, 3 and 4, and knows how to use them to plan the critique. It also shows a balance between theory and practice and plans to incorporate the writer's experience on clinical placement.

Activity 2.3

This is a good example of an introduction of an article review. It states both the topic of the article and the purpose of the review. It also mentions the audience of the article and the assumptions the writer has made about them. It describes the journal as an appropriate forum for the article, which is described as an empirical article. However, there is no information about the journal volume and issue, and no page numbers for the article.

Activity 2.5

Read these two short texts. One is more descriptive than the other. Decide which is which, and think of reasons to justify your choice.

Text 2 is more descriptive. It just presents a list of facts: having to make decisions, benefits of staying in the same room, locations of nurses' stations and patient privacy.

Chapter 3

Activity 3.2

The writer positions him/herself as an objective outsider, focusing on the studies, and programmes and their results. He/she agrees with some aspects of the studies mentioned but also indicates some of their shortcomings (e.g. 'This seems to indicate that smoking cessation in pregnancy is unsuccessful because…'). The writer uses a variety of verbs to indicate endorsement or the lack of it (e.g. 'suggest', 'seem to', 'forcefully concluded', 'should'). He/she presents the arguments that will later be challenged, but doesn't provide a transition such as 'however'. Instead, there is a suggestion that these studies indicate that support has been unsuccessful.

In this part of the text, the writer refers to previous arguments upon which the new arguments are built. However, no new evidence to support his/her points is being presented. It is difficult to judge at this point, though, the balance in the arguments as well as the logical relationship between the different parts of the argument.

The presentation of the arguments follows a logical order and this helps the writer's aim to convince the reader, but it may be, again, too early to say.

Activity 3.3

1. Maslin-Prothero is affiliated with a university in the UK, has edited several books and is a regular contributor to various journals. The text is published in association with the Royal College of Nursing in the UK. It was edited a long time ago, but a second edition has been recently published. Its intended audience is mainly student nurses and it covers most of the documents they need for their studies.

2. The authors of this research report are all affiliated with a university in the UK, and most of them have previously published in other international journals. The report was recently published (2005) and its contents follows the typical layout of a research report. It presents evidence that shows the benefits and the shortcomings of postpartum smoking cessation interventions based on the Transtheoretical Model (TTM).

3. Purdue University is a well-known and prestigious university in the USA. Their online writing lab has been created to help students improve their academic skills. The faculty in charge of developing the materials are all qualified and experienced teachers. The materials are quite varied and cover most aspects students may need for the development of their academic skills.

4. Spiegel's text is a classical reference in psychopharmacology. This is its 4th edition. Spiegel is a senior industrial pharmacologist and is affiliated with a university in Switzerland. The author's contributions are well-know in the field.

Chapter 4

Activity 4.1

Experience	Description	Reflection
Discontinue breastfeeding	Visit to the client's house The client's house Client's anxiety and reasons for it What the student midwife did What the midwife did	Client's need for information to make informed decisions Realizing the importance of consistent supervision and advice

Activity 4.2

Read the following conclusion that has been written following the outline above. Has the conclusion been developed in an effective way? Be prepared to give reasons to support your answer.

In general it is a good conclusion. However, it could be improved if the writer made it more balanced by adding something about the other skills discussed in the introduction and the body of the reflective essay. Also, the conclusion would need to specify the course of action for the needs identified in the body paragraphs.

Chapter 5

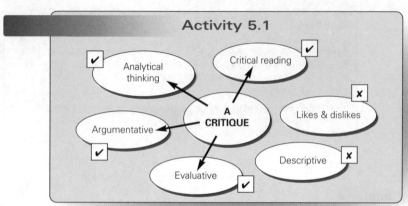

Activity 5.1

- Analytical thinking ✔
- Critical reading ✔
- A CRITIQUE
- Likes & dislikes ✘
- Argumentative ✔
- Descriptive ✘
- Evaluative ✔

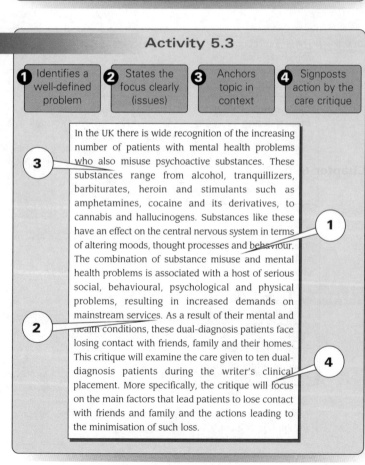

Activity 5.3

1 Identifies a well-defined problem **2** States the focus clearly (issues) **3** Anchors topic in context **4** Signposts action by the care critique

In the UK there is wide recognition of the increasing number of patients with mental health problems who also misuse psychoactive substances. These **3** substances range from alcohol, tranquillizers, barbiturates, heroin and stimulants such as amphetamines, cocaine and its derivatives, to cannabis and hallucinogens. Substances like these have an effect on the central nervous system in terms **1** of altering moods, thought processes and behaviour. The combination of substance misuse and mental health problems is associated with a host of serious social, behavioural, psychological and physical problems, resulting in increased demands on mainstream services. As a result of their mental and **2** health conditions, these dual-diagnosis patients face losing contact with friends, family and their homes. This critique will examine the care given to ten dual-diagnosis patients during the writer's clinical **4** placement. More specifically, the critique will focus on the main factors that lead patients to lose contact with friends and family and the actions leading to the minimisation of such loss.

Activity 5.4

Read the following example of a conclusion of a critique that examines the care provided to a woman in the third stage of labour. Considering what you have learnt about conclusions so far, how effective do you think this conclusion is? Give reasons for your answer.

This conclusion starts in a very effective way. It restates the identification of the main problem emerging from the care analysed and summarizes the main issues. However, in its last part it starts adding new issues that have not been mentioned before. This is exactly what conclusions should NOT do.

Activity 5.5

The recommendations made are appropriate to the topic examined. They have also indirectly revisited the weaknesses of the care critiqued, and made a point of how to solve this problem.

Chapter 6

Activity 6.1

Analyse the following statements and decide whether they are claims stating opinions (OP) or facts (FA). Be prepared to support your choices.

1 OP. It offers no support for the claims made.

2 FA. It uses references from the existing literature to support the claim made.

3 OP. It offers no support for the claims made.

4 OP. It offers no support for the claims made.

Activity 6.2

Topic: Risk assessment scales for preventing pressure ulcers

Argument A (*For*):	**Argument B** (*Against*):
Strengths	*Weaknesses*

– been developed since 1960s
– variety of instruments
– statistical comparison of
  different scales
	– 'true' sensitivity of any RAS
	  cannot be measured when
	  preventive interventions are
	  initiated

Activity 6.3

1 *Many professionals*: Who? How many?
2 *Results of research in midwifery care are inconclusive*: what results? Of what previous research?
3 *It has, for example, been suggested*: By whom? When? Where?
4 *Health promotion programmes*: Examples at the national level? Examples at the local levels?

References needed to be able to answer all these questions

Activity 6.4

A statement of the topic (1), Argument or arguments that contradict the thesis (2), A transitional marker marking a contradiction (3), Statement of the thesis (4)

Text 1
The debate surrounding evidence-based practice and the implementation of research-based knowledge in practice is well rehearsed. Some of the key issues discussed have been perceived as barriers to the implementation of knowledge, with Funk *et al.*, (1991) developing a 'barriers to research utilisation' questionnaire that has been widely adopted in the National Health Service (Retsas, 2000; Closs *et al.*, 2000; Parahoo, 2000) (**1**). However (**3**), these barriers have been mostly framed as individual responsibility – the lack of skill in research critique, the lack of interest in accessing the written knowledge base, the lack of compliance with the evidence (Kaluzny *et al.*, 1995; French, 1996) (**2**). (Clarke & Wilcockson, 2002: 397)
No statement of thesis made (**4**)

Text 2

While (**3**) in recent years there has been an increase in the number of studies examining occupational stress among community mental health nurses (Harper & Minghella, 1997; McLeod, 1997; Coffey, 1999; Drake & Brumblecombe, 1999; Burnard *et al.*, 2000) (**1**), the experiences of staff in acute inpatient settings, providing 24-hour care for people with serious mental illness, have received less attention (**2**). An investigation of acute mental health nursing commissioned for the United Kingdom's (UK) Department of Health (Higgins et al., 1997) has highlighted the need for further research in this area (**4**). (Jenkins & Elliot, 2004: 623)

Activity 6.5

Version 2

It is possible, *however*, that the differences seen are not *entirely* explainable by disappointment with the care-giver assignment. *Staniszewka and Ahmed (1999) point out* that patients' expectations are influenced by their awareness of what they *might* realistically expect. Evaluation of a service is also influenced by beliefs about the duty the service owes the client and whether or not there were circumstances outside the service's control that affected the care (*Williams et al.*, 1998). If expectations are a determinant of satisfaction with care, *it is possible that* there would have been less difference between the satisfaction scores of the two groups since women have different expectations for doctors than they do for midwives. (Harvey *et al.*, 2002: 266)

Chapter 7

Activity 7.1

Patient's name	Mrs. M	
Medical record number	ICD-9-CM 348.1	
Room number	231	
Date	18.07.06	
Problem	Description	Goal
Loss of self-image and self-esteem.	Patient presents severe loss of self-esteem due to chemotherapy.	Will regain some self-image and self-esteem in 20 days.
Approach	Assessment	Review (re-evaluation)
Encourage patient to gradually return to normal activities.	Assessment in 21 days.	After first assessment.

Activity 7.2

Text 1 is part of the introduction of the report, and Text 2 is the abstract.

Chapter 8

Activity 8.1

Text 2 shows more variation. Not all its sentences start the same way and it shows a combination of short, simple and more complex sentences.

Nurses can work in many health care settings, <u>which gives them</u> the opportunity to gain experience in all aspects of caring for clients and their families. Nurses can thus build their professional career in many different ways. <u>For instance, *they*</u> may choose to become clinical specialists or consultant nurses, or they can opt for managerial positions as a head of nursing services or supervisor of other nurses. <u>For the more academic oriented ones</u>, there are also opportunities in education and research. <u>These are just a few</u> examples of the opportunities that nurses currently have to develop their professional interests.

Activity 8.2

Cutting and repairing an episiotomy, and repairing vaginal/perineal lacerations were each proposed and retained as basic skills. *Repairing a cervical laceration* was proposed and retained as an additional skill. *There is* considerable Grade I evidence that avoiding episiotomy enhances both short- and long-term perineal integrity, supporting the midwifery philosophy of non-intervention. *This evidence* is counterbalanced by other Grade I evidence that restricting the use of episiotomy increases the risk of anterior perineal trauma.

Activity 8.3

As pressure to control hospital costs has intensified, the need to deliver the best nursing care in the most economical way has grown. Internationally research reviews show the benefits of home care. <u>For example</u>, dialysis patients can be reunited with their families and hospital beds used only when really necessary. <u>In addition</u>, by reducing hospital stays, governments undoubtedly save thousands of dollars. <u>Nevertheless</u>, it is not possible for professionals and policy-makers to estimate the resource implications of in-home services in Hong Kong unless systematic research is undertaken. (Luk, 2002: 269)

Activity 8.4

Text 1
This seems to indicate that to be effective smoking cessation intervention should consider both the fetus and the mother. **Summarize**

Text 2
To provide client-centred care, nurses should recognize culture-sensitive practices and their relation to social cultures. **Mark a transition**

Activity 8.5

Text 1
<u>In contrast to this prevailing view of women as objects</u>, many international leaders and agencies have taken action to promote women as persons with full human rights, beginning with the female child. (Thompson, 2002: 189)

Text 2
Psychiatric and Social Work pre-admission assessment have long-standing histories as requirements of UK Mental Health Acts (1983). Pre-admission nursing assessment has no such obvious legal authority; however, the practice is commonplace for most, if not all, Medium and High Security Hospitals.
   <u>Despite the widespread nature of this practice</u>, preadmission nursing assessments have received little descriptive or research attention in forensic mental health. (Watt *et al.*, 2003: 645)

Text 3
The women in the midwifery group were seen by an obstetrician during their initial visit to the midwives' clinic and at 36 weeks gestation to confirm their low-risk status.
   <u>Apart from the two mandatory obstetrician visits</u>, the midwives made autonomous decisions on the care they provided. They made referrals to, or consulted with, obstetricians and other health team members when the need arose. (Harvey *et al.*, 2002:262)

Chapter 9

Activity 9.1

Text 1
This text plagiarizes the original one by using practically the same ideas and words. Also, it claims that 'Several studies have suggested...' but it gives evidence of only two.

Text 2
This text correctly cites the information in the original text using different words. In other words, it doesn't plagiarize.

Text 3
This text not only plagiarizes the original one by using practically the same words, but also quotes the original texts incorrectly.

Activity 9.2

In general terms, it could be said that text 2 presents a better version of a re-definition. However, it can also be said that there was actually no need to redefine Chlamydia in the first place.

Activity 9.3

Lifted version
A funded pilot programme in midwifery support in a community where this support was not available provided the authors an excellent opportunity to compare this service with that of existing maternity services for women at low obstetric risk. One of the major concerns in the region, probably as a result of not having this kind of care before, related to safety.

Improved version
Harvey *et al.* (2002) compare the quality of the service provided to low risk women by existing maternity services and a new midwifery pilot programme. As midwifery services were not previously available, it was felt that the safety of the new practice should be given top priority.

Chapter 10

Activity 10.1

Text A: Anchoring the text in the field

Text B: Supporting ideas

Text C: Building an argument

Activity 10.2

Text 1: Critical stance

Text 2: Scaffolding

Activity 10.3

Reference 1 (Philips P. & Joanne Labrow, 1998): has included the authors' name initial and name. This is incorrect, as in-text references should only show surname(s).

Reference 2 (Rassool, 2001, pp.110): has used the abbreviated form for pages (pp.) rather than the one for page (p.).

Reference 3 (www.mind.org.uk): has incorrectly included the webpage rather than the name of the page (Mind, National Association for Mental Health, 2006).

Activity 10.4

Courtenay, M. 2002. Movement and mobility in R. Hogston and P. M. Simpson (Eds.): *Foundations of nursing practice*, 262–285. Basingstoke: Palgrave.

Year of publication should be given in brackets. The same holds for page numbers which should be preceded by pp.

Johnson, T and W. Taylor. (2005). *Skills for midwifery practice*. Second edn. London: Churchill Livingstone.

Jasper, M. (2003). *Beginning reflective practice: Foundations in nursing and health care*. Cheltenham: Nelson Thornes.

Savage, T. A. (2005). How do we handle conflicts with parents over unsafe oral feedings? *Rehabilitation Nursing*, 30, (pp. 7–8).

Page numbers should not be given in brackets.

References

Aston J., E. Shi, H. Bullôt, R. Galway and J. Crisp (2006) 'Quantitative evaluation of regular morning meetings aimed at improving work practices associated with effective interdisciplinary communication', *International Journal of Nursing Practice*, vol. 12: 57–63.

Atkins, S. and K. Murphy (1993) 'Reflection: a review of the literature', *Journal of Advanced Nursing*, vol. 18: 1188–92.

Buzan, T. (1991) *The Mind Map Book*. New York: Penguin.

Clarke, C.L. and J. Wilcockson (2002) 'Seeing need and developing care: exploring knowledge for and from practice', *International Journal of Nursing* Studies, vol. 39: 397–406.

Cottrell, S. (2005) *Critical Thinking Skills. Developing Effective Analysis and Argument. Basingstoke*: Palgrave Macmillan.

Davis, E. (2004) *Heart & Hands: A Midwife's Guide to Pregnancy and Birth*, 4th edn. Berkeley, CA: Celestial Arts.

Durgahee, T. (1996) 'Promoting reflection in post-graduate nursing: A theoretical model', *Nurse Education Today*, vol. 16: 419–26.

Gibbs, G. (1988) *Learning by Doing. A guide to teaching and learning methods*. Further education unit, Oxford: Oxford Polytechnic.

Harvey, S., D. Rach, M.C. Stainton, J. Jarrell and R. Brant (2002) 'Evaluation of satisfaction with midwifery care', *Midwifery*, vol. 18: 260–7.

Health Encyclopaedia, NHS Direct, available athttp://www.nhsdirect. nhs.uk/articles/alphaindex.aspx, last retrieved 9 June 2006.

Jenkins, R. and P. Elliott (2004) 'Stressors, burnout and social support: nurses in acute mental health settings', *Journal of Advanced Nursing*, 48: 622–31.

Johns, C. (2004) *Becoming a Reflective Practitioner*. Oxford: Blackwell Publishers.

Luk, Suet-Ching W. (2002) 'The home care experience as perceived by the caregivers of Chinese dialysis patients', *International Journal of Nursing Studies*, vol. 39: 269–277.

Maughan, K., B. Heyman and M. Matthews (2002) 'In the shadow of risk. How men cope with a partner's gynaecological cancer', *International Journal of Nursing Studies*, vol. 39: 27–34.

Norberg, A., E. Melin and K. Asplund (2003) 'Reactions to music, touch and object presentation in the final stage of dementia: an exploratory study', *International Journal of Nursing Studies*, vol. 40: 473–9.

Oshima, A. and A. Hogue (1998) *Writing Academic English*, 3rd edn. London: Longman.

Papanikolaou, P., M. Clark, and P.A. Lynea (2002) 'Improving the accuracy of pressure ulcer risk calculators: some preliminary evidence', *International Journal of Nursing Studies*, vol. 39: 187–94.

Rolfe, G., D. Freshwater and M. Jasper (2001) *Critical Reflection for Nurses and the Caring Professions: A users guide*. Basingstoke: Palgrave.

Schon, D.A. (1987) *Educating the Reflective Practitioner: Towards a New Design for Teaching and Learning in the Professions*. San Francisco: Jossey-Bass.

Swales, J. and C.B. Feak (1994) *Academic Writing for Graduate Students*. Ann Arbor: University of Michigan Press.

The Purdue University Online Writing Lab, available at http://owl.english. purdue.edu, last retrieved 2 June 2006.

Thompson, J.E. (2002) 'Midwives and human rights: dream or reality?' *Midwifery*, vol. 18: 188–92.

Tsaya, S.-T. and M.-L. Chen (2003) 'Acupressure and quality of sleep in patients with end-stage renal disease – a randomized controlled trial', *International Journal of Nursing Studies*, vol. 40: 1–7.

Tummers, G.E.R., G.G. van Merode and J.A. Landeweerd (2002) 'The diversity of work: differences, similarities and relationships concerning characteristics of the organisation, the work and psychological work reactions in intensive care and non-intensive care nursing', *International Journal of Nursing Studies*, vol. 39: 841–55.

Van Manen, M. (1977) 'Linking ways of knowing to ways of being practical', *Curriculum Inquiry*, 6: 205–28.

Watt, A., B. Topping-Morris, T. Mason and P. Rogers (2003) 'Pre-admission nursing assessment in a Welsh medium secure unit (1991–2000): Part 1 – an analysis of practice and cost', *International Journal of Nursing Studies*, vol. 40: 645–55.

What is Plagiarism?, Turnitin.com, available at: http://www.turnitin.com/ research_site/e_what_is_plagiarism.html, last retrieved 2 June 2006.

Widmark, C., C. Tishelman and B. Ahlberg (2002) 'A study of Swedish midwives' encounters with infibulated African women in Sweden', *Midwifery*, vol. 18: 113–25.

Index